THE BROKEN BOY

THE
BROKEN BOY

Patrick Cockburn

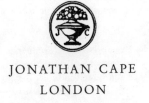

JONATHAN CAPE
LONDON

Published by Jonathan Cape 2005

2 4 6 8 10 9 7 5 3 1

Copyright © Patrick Cockburn 2005

Patrick Cockburn has asserted his right under the Copyright, Designs
and Patents Act 1988 to be identified as the author of this work

First published in Great Britain in 2005 by
Jonathan Cape
Random House, 20 Vauxhall Bridge Road, London SW1V 2SA

Random House Australia (Pty) Limited
20 Alfred Street, Milsons Point, Sydney,
New South Wales 2061, Australia

Random House New Zealand Limited
18 Poland Road, Glenfield,
Auckland 10, New Zealand

Random House South Africa (Pty) Limited
Endulini, 5A Jubilee Road, Parktown 2193, South Africa

The Random House Group Limited Reg. No. 954009
www.randomhouse.co.uk

A CIP catalogue record for this book is available from the British Library

ISBN 0-224-07108-4

Papers used by Random House are natural,
recyclable products made from wood grown in sustainable forests;
the manufacturing processes conform to the environmental
regulations of the country of origin

Typeset by Palimpsest Book Production Limited,
Polmont, Stirlingshire
Printed and bound in Great Britain by
William Clowes Ltd, Beccles, Suffolk

For Janet, Henry and Alexander

List of Illustrations

Illustration no. 19 is reproduced courtesy of the *Irish Examiner*

One

It is very easy to get polio.

I was six when I woke up with a headache and a sore throat in my bedroom in Brook Lodge, a crumbling Georgian mansion overlooking the Blackwater valley in County Cork. My forehead felt hot and the sheets were damp from sweat. My mother, Patricia Cockburn, took my temperature and asked Paddy McMahon, an elderly man who looked after the walled garden and our small herd of sheep, to bicycle into the town of Youghal a mile and a half away, to get a doctor. We owned no car and Paddy had been driving me in a horse and trap to the Loreto convent, a red-brick building on a hill overlooking Youghal bay, where the nuns were slowly teaching me to read and write. There was no phone in the house because, as my father Claud Cockburn said, it had 'blown down in a financial blizzard, some years before'.[1]

Dr John Gowen, a neatly dressed handsome man originally from England with a small practice in Youghal, arrived in his car at Brook Lodge two hours later. My mother had drawn the heavy mauve curtains across the

1

windows and I was lying in the dark. On the white-painted ceiling high above I could see the brown stains where water had found its way in past winters through cracks in the nineteenth-century lead roof and had dripped into buckets and bowls hastily placed on the floor. I was excited by the tapping sound of the water falling into the metal pails. Dr Gowen gently asked me about my headache and told me to roll up my pyjama jacket so he could listen to my chest with his stethoscope. I liked the feel of cold metal against my skin. He had treated me a year before when my mother had accidentally driven a garden fork through my toe when I was standing next to her, my wellington boots covered by earth, when she was planting strawberries in the garden. Dr Gowen later told me that he found me shy and difficult to talk to, but if I appeared timid to him it was because I was not used to dealing with people apart from my family and the three servants: Paddy, my nanny Kitty Lee, and Norah Maloney, a cheerful woman who lived on a farm in the hills behind Brook Lodge.[2]

The first signs of illness had appeared the previous day. Kitty had taken me for a walk to Youghal to visit my first cousin Shirley Arbuthnot, one year older than me, who lived in Myrtle Grove, a Tudor mansion within the ancient town walls where my mother had grown up. Sir Walter Ralegh had lived there briefly in the late sixteenth century. I had been told – and it is the sort of graphic tale that adults suppose will amuse children – it was here beneath the four giant yew trees outside the house, so old that their gnarled dark brown branches had grown into each other, that Ralegh had smoked the first pipe of tobacco in Europe. A maid, thinking the great explorer was on fire, had hurled a bucket of water over him. I was less interested in Ralegh than in using the swing which hung from one of the yew branches and playing with Shirley. But she had gone for a walk with her nanny and was nowhere to be found. Her mother Rosemary was there and noticed that I looked feverish. She put me and Kitty in her car, an elderly vehicle with wooden slats on the sides, and drove us back to Brook Lodge.[3] My mother was very worried, though she did not send Paddy for the doctor until the next morning. She got a friend to phone my father, who was still in London, simply saying I was ill. He heard the telephone ringing as he returned to the house at 9.30 p.m. The message did not say exactly what was wrong with me but it did not have to. He immediately flew to Dublin, hired a car to drive the couple of hundred miles to Youghal and arrived home just before the doctor appeared.[4]

It did not take Dr Gowen long to diagnose why I was sick. A polio epidemic had started three months before, in early July 1956, in Cork city thirty miles away. I had the symptoms. They were little different from those of flu, with a headache, sweating, rapid pulse and vomiting. An ambulance was called. It was a cream-coloured vehicle which stopped beside the tall green yew trees on the drive outside the enormous drawing-room windows, which rose fifteen feet from the ground at the front of the house. I was crying as I was carried from my room on the second floor, down the elegant but rickety staircase and through the long dark hall on to the front lawn. My mother, Kitty and Norah, all in tears, were waiting by the open rear doors of the ambulance as the ambulance men, dressed in white coats, laid me on a stretcher inside. My mother, searching desperately for something comforting to say that would cheer me up, said: 'The driver will turn on the siren and all the other cars will have to get out of the way.' I was not comforted. I sensed the anxiety of the people standing looking at me. 'I don't want him to sound the horn! I don't want it!' I cried and sobbed louder.

I was extremely frightened in the back of the ambulance. I had been driven to Cork before but I was always sitting upright on the back seat. Lying down I could only see, through the rear windows, the feathery leaves on the top branches of trees beside the road and the upper storeys of the higher buildings in Youghal and the four villages we drove through – Killeagh, Castlemartyr, Midleton and Carrigtohill – before we reached the outskirts of Cork city. Over the next few years I became used to travelling on this road lying flat on my back and I came to know exactly where we were from such glimpses, but this first time I found it strange and upsetting.

I had spent most of my time with Kitty Lee. I thought of my mother as a friendly but more distant presence. Kitty first came to Brook Lodge, after some months looking after my grandmother Olive Arbuthnot at Myrtle Grove, before I was born. My first memory of any kind is of lying as a baby in my pram, as raindrops splashed on the hood, and seeing Kitty looking down at me. She was a short strong woman, then in her early forties, the right half of her face covered with a large purple birthmark. Bessie O'Callaghan, Shirley's nanny and Kitty's best friend, told me: 'You were her whole life. She forgot the older boys when you were along.'[5] She had a deeply affectionate nature, was highly intelligent and had a natural authority in dealing with children and adults, whom she treated exactly alike. She was religious, as was everybody else in Youghal, but her affliction – she had also lost the sight of one eye in an accident at the age of eleven – gave her a great ability to endure and overcome suffering. She was also strongly nationalist. One day – it must have been my first visit to England when I was about five – when we were walking on the stony beach at Brighton, where I liked to visit a toy bear in a glass case on the pier who drank a glass of beer when a penny was put in a slot, she warned me: 'Don't talk so loud. The English are listening.' I regarded them with deeper suspicion than before. Her animosities were gentle if unyielding. She spent almost all her life in Youghal, where she had been born and knew everybody. When she was not living in Brook Lodge she bicycled to the house from Youghal every day.

I never thought about the purple birthmark because I was used to it from the time I was a baby. Kitty slept in my room until I was four and almost never left my side when I was awake. I lived mostly in the nursery beside my bedroom and in the kitchen where there were always people to talk to. My father had once told Kitty to put some loose change left by a departed guest in my money box. Ever afterwards she considered that I had a feudal right to any money momentarily placed in view. My black tin money box, kept in a chest of drawers in my bedroom, was soon too small to contain the large Irish pennies with a hen engraved on one side. Also in the box, though never as many as I wanted, were florins with a leaping salmon and half-crowns with a strong-looking horse. Every few months we would visit the post office in Youghal to have additional cash confiscated by Kitty placed in my account. I was prohibited by the Post Office from taking out the money until I was seven, which I therefore thought of as an age of responsibility and maturity frustratingly far in the future.

The journey in that ambulance was the first time that I was truly alone. It took me to St Finbarr's, the fever hospital, a converted stone nineteenth-century workhouse, built at the time of the Irish Famine on the south side of Cork. I was admitted on 30 September 1956 according to the hospital register.[6] The first death in the epidemic, a girl of five called Kay Long, had occurred there six weeks earlier. It had happened before doctors in Cork had come to recognise that her flu-like symptoms might have a more sinister cause and the polio virus had not been diagnosed. She died soon after she said she felt ill.[7]

I did not know it but ever since the first six victims had been diagnosed with polio in early July of that year, St Finbarr's had been regarded with terror by people in Cork. They crossed the road outside to avoid walking close to its walls for fear of infection. It was widely believed that the authorities were lying about the death rate and bodies were being smuggled out through a back door.[8] The hospital was old, but the nuns from the Order of Mercy, who were in charge, and lay nurses were friendly and kind. I was in bed in a crowded ward for three weeks. Nobody apart from the doctors and nurses was allowed in to see me for fear of infection. At the time I arrived Roman Catholic priests and Protestant clergy were permitted to visit the ward, but they too were later excluded.

I was mystified by the wire cage holding up the blankets and sheets in a mound at the lower end of my bed so they did not weigh down on my legs. Nor did I understand why the doctors, with solemn looks on their faces, would ask me once or twice a day to wiggle my toes or try to raise my legs. I was appalled by the shiny stainless-steel bedpans proffered by the nurses and I refused to use them. Eventually a brown rubber tube was produced and inserted into my bottom and I was given an enema. Every few days a nurse would point to the door of the ward and I could see my parents, with fixed, almost manic smiles, waving from the other side of a glass porthole.

A few days later I was joined by my brother Andrew. He was three years older than me and dark-haired and tall for his age while I was fair and of medium height. He had already spent one year as a boarder at St Stephen's, a Protestant school in the Dundrum district of Dublin. It was run by a generally benign but heavy-drinking former naval chaplain called Hugh Brodie and his wife Lettice. Andrew was back at St Stephen's after the summer holidays when I was taken to hospital. My father had immediately telephoned the school to tell the headmaster to send him home. Brodie, presumably knowing that his school would have to close if it was known that one of the pupils had polio, was quick to get Andrew off his hands. He was summoned to the headmaster's office. 'I was told I was ill but nobody mentioned polio,' he said. 'I had complained of back pains the day before. They must have guessed what it was but even so they did not send me to hospital but put me on the train back to Cork as soon as they could. By the time I reached Cork station I was feeling pretty bad.'[9] My father was waiting for him on the platform. He later recalled: 'I really thought that all might be well up to the very last moment when the diesel train pulled into the station and Andrew got out. I then saw that his body was bowed slightly forward in an awkward way and he was moving his legs sluggishly.'[10] The two of them drove back to Brook Lodge and Dr Gowen was once again summoned. 'It was terrifying,' he said. 'He was showing signs of nerve damage.' By the next morning Andrew had joined me in St Finbarr's. I was pleased to see him. He was in a different ward from myself, on the ground floor while I was one floor up, but a nurse gave him piggyback rides – we were not allowed to walk – up and down the stairs so he could talk to me.

I felt that something terrible and incomprehensible had happened to me, but I enjoyed being the centre of attention, the doctors gathering round my bed several times a day. I resented it later when my father, who always adopted an optimistic approach to his own frequent illnesses, said to me: 'You were lucky to get polio in an epidemic so the doctors immediately knew what was wrong with you and didn't think you had a cold.' It was believed that the polio virus destroyed more muscles if you moved around too much after you caught it. But I did not like the idea of being less unfortunate than I imagined and therefore less of an object of interest.

I was largely right in feeling uniquely unlucky. The Cork epidemic, during which at least 50,000 people got the polio virus – though a far smaller number were crippled – was one of the last great outbreaks of polio anywhere in Western Europe. An effective vaccine had been discovered, after immense scientific effort, by Dr Jonas Salk in the US in 1954. Church bells had rung out in celebration across America on 12 April 1955 when it was announced that a mass test of this vaccine showed that it worked. In the summer of 1956, as the polio virus was claiming more victims in Cork, the first emergency mass vaccination through injection was bringing to an end an epidemic in Chicago.

The new vaccine was known about in Ireland. But at this time Irish doctors did little which had not already been accepted by the medical establishment in Britain where so many of them had been trained. The nurses in St Finbarr's were offered the Salk vaccine during the summer but turned it down, after holding a meeting, from a mixture of motives. To their credit they felt that it would be wrong to accept protection against the virus which was not available to the rest of the population of Cork. Kathleen O'Callaghan, an efficient and energetic young doctor who was treating me at the time, said that 'we felt it wasn't necessary for us because we had been close to polio for so long that if we were going to get it we would have got it already. We also wondered if it might not reawaken any virus we might already have. We didn't trust the American vaccination.'[11] The latter suspicion may have been reinforced by a widely publicised disaster during the mass test of the vaccine in the US the previous year. One batch of vaccine, through some defect in its production, had contained live rather than dead virus. Some two hundred children caught the disease, many were paralysed and several died.

I am not sure what age I was when I began to feel astonished that my parents had taken myself aged six and my brother Andrew, aged nine, back to Cork two months after the epidemic had started. They knew that the other name for polio was 'infantile paralysis', because it primarily affected children. Of the first 113 confirmed cases of polio in Cork in early August, the time we returned to Brook Lodge, only five were adults.[12] Other children were being hastily evacuated from the city by their terrified parents. We had moved temporarily from Ireland to London a few months before the first cases of polio were diagnosed in Cork in early July. Three weeks later Dr Michael Goold, the head of St Finbarr's, was appealing for calm and unwisely declaring that there was no need for 'a panic reaction to the polio epidemic'.[13] This predictably increased the conviction among people in Cork, always cynical about any pronouncement by the authorities, that not only was there every reason to panic but that the true horrendous facts about the spread of polio in the city were being suppressed.

In the late spring of 1956 my parents had rented a house in Hampstead while my father was working with Malcolm Muggeridge, then recently famous as one of the first aggressive television interviewers. Muggeridge had been appointed editor of *Punch* and was making a determined effort to revive the magazine, which, its original acerbic humour long abandoned, had become highly decorous and tedious to read. Cheques from *Punch* temporarily alleviated my parents' desperate shortage of money. My father was well known, indeed notorious, but for reasons never likely to lead to a steady income. As a former communist, denounced by Senator McCarthy in the US as the eighty-fourth most dangerous Red in the world, he could seldom write under his own name. In 1954 John

Huston filmed his novel *Beat the Devil*, written under the name of James Helvick – one of four noms de plume he was then using. It starred Humphrey Bogart and Gina Lollobrigida and was fairly successful. But because of McCarthy's denunciation my father's real name could not appear on the screen, so it did us less good than he had hoped. The film rights had been sold for three thousand pounds, a sum which went a long way in Ireland in the early 1950s, but in our case not quite far enough. My father believed that by moving to Hampstead for six months he could, in addition to working for *Punch*, sell more freelance articles, seeking, he wrote, 'to shore up, and even perhaps establish on sound foundations, our always tottering financial structure'.[14]

I never liked London. The substantial house in Hampstead seemed to me poky and alien compared to Brook Lodge with its large walled garden, streams with soft mossy banks and interesting places to hide among the chestnut and sycamore trees. I enjoyed digging deep holes in the ground, far more difficult in the sticky clay of a Hampstead garden than in the dark earth at home. My mother, also, detested living in London for more than short periods. She was eager to get back to Brook Lodge where she was breeding horses for hunting, gardening and farming the four fields around the house. She had inherited a disdain, common among some of the Anglo-Irish gentry, towards the English as being both colonial oppressors and at the same time tediously bourgeois. She also, so my father believed, had another Anglo-Irish trait. Accustomed to the London social season ending in late July – though it was thirty years since she had been a debutante – she instinctively imagined 'that to be in

London in August was to indulge in a perverse form of masochism'.

In early August my parents took the disastrous decision to return to Ireland. At the last moment they hesitated. They had heard that a 'somewhat abnormal number of cases of polio had been reported in Cork city'. My father wrote later that there was also polio in London, and at least in Ireland 'we could, at home, virtually isolate the children on the farm'. This sounds like retrospective justification for a decision probably really taken by my mother, although she had received several letters from Ireland warning her not to come.

We took a train from London to Wales and then a boat to Cork. It was in the crowded bar of the *Innisfallen*, as it crossed the Irish Sea, that my father had several conversations with other passengers who expressed, he later recalled, 'the sort of apprehensions you encountered among people travelling to London during the bombing. I thought they were trying to make life more exciting.' Years later, after spending a quarter of a century working as a journalist in Belfast, Beirut, Baghdad, Jerusalem and Moscow, I came to recognise this deceptive feeling which comes from living in violent places. Because people commonly exaggerate the dangers to be faced around the next corner it is easy to discount or dismiss what they say. But every so often they are going to be right, with lethal results for oneself. If my father had not spent his formative years in Budapest, where he could see the bodies of political murder victims floating in the waters of the Danube, or in Berlin just before the rise of Hitler, he might have taken more seriously the warnings of the men drinking away their fears with glasses of whiskey and Guinness at the bar of the *Innisfallen*.

We reached Cork docks late in the morning and mountains of luggage were packed into a van. We hired a car with driver to take us to Youghal. But first we wanted to do some shopping in Patrick Street in the centre of Cork. This was normally packed with cars and people – Cork pedestrians were notoriously aggressive and hammered their fists on the bonnets of vehicles which did not stop quickly enough for them – making it impossible to park. On this day the city was agreeably empty. The same thing was true of the shops. One of us said that we seemed to have hit on a lucky day. The driver of the car turned around in astonishment. 'People are afraid,' he said. 'They're afraid to come into Cork. Business is going to hell. If the epidemic goes on, in a few weeks half the shops in this street will be bankrupt.'[15] We hastily bought a few essentials and hurried to Youghal.

It is easy to see why my parents, as we drove home, thought their house was isolated enough to escape the epidemic. There had been no case of polio in Youghal in recent months, though there had been sporadic incidents in previous years. Some children in Cork had even been sent there for safety by their parents. Very old and very beautiful, Youghal felt different from the outside world. My father, quoting with approval E. M. Forster on the poet Cavafy, said that 'it stood at an angle to the world'. It was a small place of five thousand people squeezed between the side of a long steep hill and the estuary of the Blackwater river as it enters the Atlantic. The ever-changing Irish light made the river seem to sparkle, its colour swiftly changing from blue to green and then to dark grey and black. Just before it reaches the sea the Blackwater is held back by a long low peninsula of sand

13

called the Ferry Point, sticking out from a green hill opposite the town. Behind it a broad silver lake forms at high tide, giving me the feeling that the town was an island surrounded by water.

Youghal was mostly built along two streets, one running beside the old quays and the other, the main street, running along the base of the hill. The main street was the centre of most of the town's activities, containing all its shops and most of its dark little pubs. Perhaps because Youghal had no room to expand – and for centuries its inhabitants preferred to stay safely inside its high medieval walls which still stood – the houses were pressed tightly together. The congestion so often cursed by travellers trying to pass through the town, meant the centre of Youghal was always crowded, giving a sense of warm sociability normally found only in the heart of much larger cities. Funeral processions, of which there were a great many, were always of great length, whatever the popularity of the deceased, because all the vehicles passing through the town would pile up behind the hearse as it crawled towards the cemetery beside the single remaining wall of an old abbey on the northern outskirts of town. Just off the main street was my mother's family home Myrtle Grove, the oldest unfortified large house in Ireland, protected by the massive town walls. Horsedrawn traps, gigs and carts were still common in our part of Ireland in the mid-1950s and there were two blacksmiths conveniently placed on the road to Brook Lodge. One of them had stables attached and I used to enjoy going there when we stopped at the blacksmith on our way to the bank, journeys which, given our chronic lack of money, were presumably less welcome to my parents.

On the far side of Youghal there were a couple of small modern textile factories opposite the greyhound-racing track. But once you passed them the town had changed little since the nineteenth century. It had last prospered before the Famine as a port. Ships negotiated its dangerous sandbars and mud-flats to carry goods and passengers up and down the Blackwater. But by 1956 its stately eighteenth-century stone warehouses were abandoned. Only a few small coaling vessels, reputedly supplementing their incomes by smuggling pornography, occasionally tied up beside the fishing boats along the stone quays. The most exciting event in Youghal's recent history was a tribute to its antiquity, though some of the town's more cynical inhabitants saw it as further underlining the moribund state of the local economy over the previous century. In 1954 its waterfront was used in the opening scenes of the film of *Moby Dick* because it more closely resembled a nineteenth-century New England whaling town than anything that could still be found in America.

It was hoped, though without much confidence, that the film would encourage tourists to visit. At that time there was still a railway from Cork. It ran over a bog just outside Youghal, making the carriages, much to my enjoyment the few times I was on the train, bounce up and down on the springy turf. The little station by the long sandy beach was overlooked by a hotel which, with touching honesty, was named the Railway View. It dated from the time when people were more interested in looking at a railway engine than the Atlantic. Behind the hotel was a hill with a holy well and a blackthorn bush beside it where people tied white rags after making a wish.

We reached Brook Lodge along a narrow road which climbed past the grey rock face of a disused quarry filled with dark green gorse. Once there we felt safe enough. There was a walled garden and four fields. I rode around on an elderly white donkey called Jacky. I spent days happily but ineffectively trying to dam one of the streams with pebbles and mud. We were forbidden to go to the beach in case we met infected children from Cork, but I did not mind this since I could not swim and was bored by sandcastles. I spent a lot of my time walking with our dog, a brown-and-white mongrel terrier called Charlie (after the famous eighteenth-century radical Charles James Fox), as he inspected his deposits of bones, concealed in the grass around the house. He regarded two roads which ran on either side of our land as being definitively part of his territory and objected to any other dog using them. Asserting his rights was a full-time occupation since most of the farmers travelling by Brook Lodge had one or more dogs with them. Charlie, with me in tow, would rush backwards and forwards across a field between the two roads barking and shouting canine insults at the intruders.

Brook Lodge was essentially two houses linked at one corner by doorways on both the ground and first floors. Each building expressed the political expectations, optimistic or pessimistic, of its Anglo-Irish owners at the time it was erected. The oldest part, built soon after the Elizabethan conquest, was a dour stone farmhouse with small windows, and in the courtyard, beside a shed where the gig and trap were kept, was a deep well faced with great blocks of carefully cut stone. It was not a house built by people confident in the friendliness of their neighbours. On the road outside the house was an ivy-covered guard tower, once part of the outer defences of Youghal, converted into a stable. Two hundred years after the farmhouse was built the owner, a rich but unpopular Protestant clergyman called Drew, decided that political conditions were calm enough for him to dispense with the fortifications. He built an elegant Georgian mansion with five enormous windows, fifteen foot by ten foot, giving a splendid view of the Blackwater river shimmering in the distance. Unfortunately for him he soon found, when the land wars became more intense, that his grand new windows, which filled the house with light, also made him and his family an easy target for the stones and shotguns of angry Irish tenant farmers.

Drew immediately set to work to build a fake medieval castle called Heathfield Towers two large fields away from Brook Lodge. In an era influenced by the romances of Sir Walter Scott, mock-Gothic castles were common enough in England and the less violent parts of Ireland, but the Reverend Drew's fortifications had a purely practical intention and were nothing to do with *Ivanhoe* or nostalgia for a more colourful age. His slit windows and battlements were to protect him and his sons as they fired their rifles at their attackers. As an afterthought he added a more modern wing to his newly fortified residence, and even placed the two defiant stone lions which had once stood on either side of the drive to Brook Lodge at the entrance, but his original pessimistic expectations turned out to be correct and it was soon burned to the ground, leaving the castle standing alone, its central tower rising above the trees.

My father liked this story. He enjoyed the idea of the smug and overconfident clergyman in his mansion suddenly

17

having to decamp in terror to lurk, gun at the ready, in medieval squalor in Heathfield Towers. But he himself was also, in a sense, on the run. Notorious in the thirties as the radical editor of the anti-Fascist newsletter the *Week* and as a communist, he had moved to Ireland in 1947, first staying at Myrtle Grove. He had good reason for keeping a low profile. But his withdrawal to Ireland did not reduce his notoriety. A few years after he arrived he was unexpectedly attacked by Senator McCarthy and a little later denounced by an old friend, Otto Katz, shortly before Katz was executed after a Stalinist show trial in Prague, as Colonel Cockburn of British intelligence. Several score people were arrested for having spoken to him.

Here was another reason why my parents so disastrously underestimated the threat to their children from polio. Both were used to living dangerously. My father had resigned from a well-paid and prestigious job as New York correspondent of *The Times* to start the *Week* on a capital of fifty pounds. He commanded a battalion in the Spanish Civil War after all its officers had deserted to the other side. My mother, brought up at Myrtle Grove during the Irish War of Independence, was walking with her nanny when she saw Sir Henry Wilson, the former British Chief of Staff, shot dead on his own doorstep by an IRA gunman. She had travelled through the forests of the Congo to make a language map. During the Second World War my parents' house in St John's Wood in London had been demolished by a V-1 rocket. Neither courted danger, but nor were they likely to listen to prudent counsels advising against a return to Cork during the polio epidemic.

*

My parents did not realise the danger they were heading into because – and this was true of the great majority of people in Cork during the epidemic – they did not understand the curious and implacable nature of the disease. Brook Lodge might look safe but it was, in fact, more dangerous to live behind its walls than in a tenement in the slums of Cork or Calcutta. The polio virus had never killed or crippled in the same way as other great plagues. It does not behave like typhus or cholera. It has a strange history. An ancient Egyptian stele portraying a young man with a staff and a withered right leg – looking unnervingly like my own in the years to come – is evidence that it may have existed some 3,500 years ago. It struck at individuals. Sir Walter Scott got it when he was eighteen months old and was crippled in one leg – despite his godfather's attempt to cure Scott's lameness by wrapping him in the bloody skin of a recently killed sheep.[16]

In the last two decades of the nineteenth century polio took on a new and more menacing form. It ceased to be sporadic. For the first time there were polio epidemics and they happened on a mass scale in the richer countries like the USA, Denmark, Sweden, Australia and New Zealand. This was because public health was improving, with better water supply and sewage systems. Previously people had lived in symbiosis with the polio virus. The majority of small children were self-immunised because they got the disease, often without symptoms, when they were still protected by their mothers' antibodies. The virus, located in the alimentary canal, spread easily through excreta. In the past it was only in the most isolated places that the virus could find a pool of victims without immunity large enough for it to spread in epidemic form.

The first epidemic ever described took place in the early nineteenth century in St Helena, the dreary island in the South Atlantic chosen by the victorious allies as Napoleon's final place of exile because of its extreme isolation. The event was noticed by Charles Bell, the Scottish doctor whose acute powers of observation led Arthur Conan Doyle to take him as a model on whom the character of Sherlock Holmes was partly based. Dr Bell's curiosity about the disease was aroused when he was consulted by the wife of a clergyman in St Helena about her daughter who had one wasted leg. In talking about the illness the girl's mother, so Dr Bell recorded in a lecture published in 1844, mentioned that 'an epidemic fever spread among all the children in the island about three or five years of age; her child was ill of the same fever. It was afterwards discovered that all the children who had the fever, were similarly affected with want of growth in some parts of their bodies or limbs! This deserves to be inquired into.'[17] It was of course the very remoteness of St Helena which made its children so vulnerable to the spread of the disease. They had not been exposed to the virus from an early age and therefore lacked natural immunity. If they met a carrier they would have no protection. And this they were likely to do. For every person who becomes ill because of the polio virus there are hundreds who catch the disease but show no visible symptoms or are unaware there is anything wrong with them. But while they are infected they easily pass on the disease to others.

The mystery about how polio spread and why it would strike certain individuals and families made people dread polio more than other epidemic diseases which killed in greater numbers. People were doubly frightened because the virus struck at their children and it maimed rather than killed. Its symbol was less the coffin than the wheelchair, like that of Franklin Delano Roosevelt who caught polio in 1921; the 'iron lung' to help victims to breathe; and callipers and crutches to help them walk. In the USA it became it became known as 'The Crippler' and during an epidemic in New York in 1916 there were even greater signs of panic than in Cork forty years later. Towns outside the city in Long Island and New Jersey tried to protect themselves by sending deputy sheriffs to patrol the roads armed with shotguns. They turned back all cars carrying children under the age of sixteen. Strange stories spread, such as one that blondes were more vulnerable than brunettes. Cats were suspected of spreading the disease and 72,000 of them were hunted down and killed.[18] In our house Kitty Lee always suspected that I had caught the illness from the poisonous exhalations rising from a small swamp near Brook Lodge where I liked to play. 'You were always going down to that marshy place,' she said. 'I blame it for what happened to you.'[19]

It was a very middle-class disease. Doctors began to understand that it was children from the better-off and most hygienic families who were falling ill. But this was so contrary to popular perception of epidemic disease, which associated it with poverty and dirt, that it was never really accepted. In New York it was suspected that newly arrived Italian immigrants, fresh off the boats from the slums of Naples and Palermo, must be the source of the epidemic. A century of medical propaganda had created an unbreakable connection in people's minds between

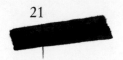

illness and lack of hygiene. Even at the age of five in my classroom in the Loreto convent, close by Youghal lighthouse, I had experienced this. I was given a green-coloured exercise book in which I painfully tried to form the letters of the alphabet. I felt bored. But I was fascinated by an improving cartoon on the back of the inside cover of the exercise book. A series of simple pictures showed evil germs, portrayed as globular and menacing, preparing to assault a child with the assistance of their friend 'dirt'. The final illustration showed them being compelled to retreat in confusion in the face of a triumphant counter-attack by the forces of soap and regular washing. I found the exact medical significance of this perplexing because I thought that 'germs' and 'Germans' were the same thing, both of whom, in those early post-war years, I had heard being ill-spoken of at home.

If the isolation of Brook Lodge had been complete, as my father and mother believed, we still might have escaped infection. But, in returning to Ireland, my father had agreed that he would continue to work for *Punch* one week in three. He would take the train from Cork to Dublin, then the site of the nearest airport, before flying on to London. He badly needed the money. Polio was not the only threat on the horizon. When my mother and he had moved into Brook Lodge my mother said the house had bailiffs like other houses had mice. Their finances had improved a little but they now had two sons at private schools. The friendly local writ server appeared with unnerving regularity at the front door. After a few minutes' amicable conversation he would quietly press a piece of paper into my father's hand which demanded his appearance in court to explain why he had not paid some long-overdue bill.

My father went to London two or three times in August and early September. On one train to Dublin he noticed that Dubliners, who had been compelled to travel to Cork on business, were visibly trying not to associate with Cork people if they could possibly avoid it. He observed, perhaps not with sufficient alarm, that Dubliners would nervously shuffle down to the other end of the carriage on hearing a Cork accent. He recalled that people from Cork found themselves 'without the slightest word being said – and perhaps with not much of a conscious thought being thought – sitting at one end of the bar and buffet car, with the Dubliners at the other'.[20]

The Dubliners were right to be anxious. At about this time my father suffered a severe headache and a pricking feeling in the tips of his fingers. My eldest brother Alexander felt the same thing. Both at first dismissed this as meaningless. Doctors later told my father that the headache with the pricking of the fingertips was a symptom of polio. He had no further illness but, if he had indeed got polio, he had become a carrier, making it likely that on his return to Brook Lodge where, like the children of St Helena, we had no immunity, the rest of us would catch the disease.

Two

Before Aids the disease which most terrified people was polio. By the time I was being driven from Brook Lodge to St Finbarr's panic had spread through Cork. People from the city were being treated as pariahs in the rest of the country. A letter signed 'People of Dublin', sent to the Minister of Health in early August, a month after the epidemic had started, conveys a sense of growing hysteria. The writer was enraged that people from Cork were being allowed to enter Dublin in their thousands to attend a hurling match in Croke Park. He or she angrily demanded that they be stopped. 'Let Cork's own people keep their Polio and not infect our clean city,' the letter concludes. 'Wake up and do something before the Polio of the Corkonians is laid upon us.'[1]

The health authorities believed they must do everything possible to prevent mass panic. They wanted schools and colleges to open for the new academic year and sports fixtures to go ahead as arranged before the epidemic. But the tactic of playing down the seriousness of the outbreak proved counter-productive. Too many people saw it as proof that government officials were wilfully blind to the threat from the disease. Anonymous letters, pleading or enraged, sent to the Department of Health at the height of the summer reflect the terror felt in the city far better than the deliberately bland and comforting newspaper headlines suggesting that everything was under control. A letter, ungrammatical and written in block capitals, arrived at the end of August from 'worried fathers and mothers'. They begged the government to stop children from the Cork area, potential carriers of the disease, returning to schools and colleges in the rest of the country:

> We parents are terrified! We have no farm or shops to leave to our children – just depending on wages and salary. Those who have farms etc. are secure enough to provide for such victims. We are not rich enough to send them further afield. We have no choice but to send them back to these colleges etc. – from which they hope to be able to earn their daily bread later on. So please don't blame us for being worried. This terrifying sickness seems to be creeping along.[2]

Another letter requests 'all the boarding schools in Co. Cork to be closed for a time until this plague of polio disappears'.[3]

My father had observed passengers on the train from Cork to Dublin scurrying nervously away from people with a Cork accent. Travellers from Cork faced further problems when they reached the capital. Danny Murphy, then a twenty-year-old lorry driver, had difficulty finding a bed for the night in Dublin. 'When they saw you were from Cork they didn't want you. They were all terrified.'[4]

John Creedon from West Cork, who caught polio at this time, recalls with retrospective glee that his parents' house was on a road and other farmers would walk through muddy fields rather than come close to it. 'They wouldn't even pass the house. There was a fierce scare. They couldn't even get their milk to the creamery.'[5]

Goods as well as people from Cork were suspect. The manager of a furnishing company called Murdoch's from Bray, south of Dublin, wrote to the Health Ministry explaining that within seven days he expected a consignment of pottery to arrive from Carrigaline in Cork. He politely asked 'whether you would advise delaying delivery of these goods in view of the present polio epidemic in the area. We understand that this pottery would be packed in straw.' The ministry equivocated and then advised him to accept the pottery.[6]

Officials in the Department of Health were edgy about telling enquirers how to react to the epidemic. Their responses were often evasive and contradictory. Diplomats at the Irish embassy in London said they had heard a rumour, widespread among Irish immigrants, that the Irish government was about to introduce a ban on ships visiting Cork. The embassy noted with exasperation that it had no information about the epidemic other than what appeared in the papers. It needed to know if it should encourage or discourage people, either immigrants returning from holiday or tourists, from visiting the city. The diplomats said many people from Cork had already cancelled their annual holidays or were about to do so.[7] Health officials in Dublin drafted a peculiarly slippery reply, saying that the Minister of Health believed the epidemic to be 'mild' and there was 'no need for public alarm'. In a sentence of contorted prose, perhaps unconsciously reflecting their own hidden fears, the officials said: 'In view of the Minister's statement regarding the nature of the epidemic it would seem that persons having business in the Cork area need not refrain from visiting there.' They then go on to cover themselves further by adding that 'in the case of others, however, it would be prudent that any unnecessary travelling to the area should be deferred'.[8]

These equivocations infuriated many people. In another letter a mother denounced the Minister of Health T. F. O'Higgins for simultaneously opposing unnecessary travel – thereby implying there was a risk of catching polio and possibly being crippled for life – and allowing thousands of people from Cork to visit Dublin for a hurling match. 'I think it was disgraceful of you to expose the children and people of Dublin to such danger,' continued the writer. 'If there is an outbreak in the next few weeks you will be responsible and have it on your conscience – but it will be us mothers who will have the anxiety and sorrow if our children are struck down and I hope you will remember this.'[9]

The local political leaders on Cork Corporation generally followed the doctors in saying that everything possible was being done to stop the spread of polio. Only occasionally did the mask slip and they acknowledged the fear in their city which my parents and I had witnessed in the empty streets of Cork when we arrived on board the *Innisfallen* in early August. A week earlier, on 24 July, John Bermingham, an influential member of the Corporation, had suddenly denounced the local doctors in charge of combating the epidemic. He was annoyed by the failure of Jack Saunders, the hard-working and authoritarian doctor who was the Medical Officer of Health of the city, to turn up at a meeting of the Corporation. Suddenly squeaks of fear become audible in the Council room. Berminghan said he 'was afraid the public had lost confidence in the public health authority of the Corporation'. He excused himself by saying that he was only reflecting what people were saying on the streets. Another Council member added that 'the feeling in the city was seeping into the Council itself'.[10]

The officials in the Department of Health had, if they had dared use it, a perfectly good defence for their action or inaction. They could have admitted that there was very little they or anybody else could do to stop the spread of the epidemic. They knew in detail about its progress because doctors in St Finbarr's were under strict orders to telephone Dublin every morning at 9 a.m. to tell them about the number of new victims.[11] There was nothing to be done except wait for the disease to burn itself out, but it was impolitic to admit to impotence in the face of the threat too loudly or too frequently. Some senior doctors in Cork pointed this out. Dr Gerald McCarthy, the Medical Officer of Health for the county, wrote testily to the Chief Medical Adviser to the Health Department in Dublin saying that restrictions on Cork people 'are, in my opinion, unduly strict, and in any case they are quite nonsensical'. No attempt to quarantine the city could have any effect while the main railway line and road linking Cork and Dublin remained open, carrying thousands of people like my father between the two cities. Dr McCarthy wrote: 'If I had my way, apart from isolating in hospital every case detected in its early stages, I would

29

take no other elaborate precautions.'[12] Doctors and nurses at St Finbarr's were not banned from visiting the rest of Cork but they kept out of restaurants and went to Mass in a church in the grounds of the hospital.

Pauline Kent, a committed and hard-working young blonde physiotherapist from Fermoy, a market town on the upper reaches of the Blackwater, was exercising polio victims in the hope that they could regain the use of their muscles if there was still a flicker of life in them. Many years before in the 1930s her eleven-year-old sister had died, her breathing paralysed by the virus, five days after being first diagnosed with polio. Pauline discovered early on in the epidemic that she and everybody else from Cork were regarded with real fear in the rest of Ireland. On 31 August 1956, a month or so before I caught the illness, an elderly relative of Pauline's called Giacomo Roche, a venerable figure who had been Roman Catholic bishop of Cloyne in east Cork for over thirty years, died of old age. Then as now it was almost impossible in Ireland not to attend the funeral of a family member or close friend whatever the difficulties or dangers. 'Our relatives came from all parts of the country to his funeral,' she recalled in an irritated tone. 'But they were more frightened of the living than the dead. They knew that I treated polio victims. They would not stand near me and my mother by the graveside. My mother had prepared a meal for fifteen members of the family. But as soon as the service was over they were all making excuses and jumping back into their cars so there was nobody to eat the food. My mother was very upset.'[13]

Surprisingly, not everybody tried to avoid catching

polio. Kathleen O'Callaghan, one of the most capable doctors in St Finbarr's, talked to some parents who prayed that, if polio was to strike their family, it would affect them and not their children. They therefore took no precautions, useless though those would probably have been, to avoid catching it. There was no belief, as there was during the great plagues of the Middle Ages, that the epidemic was a divine punishment being visited on the people of Cork for their sins. But there was a feeling that the disease had to be accepted as God's will and it would be wrong to rail against fate. Dr McCarthy had from the start of the epidemic been issuing statements which he presumably thought would reassure the population. It is easy to see why, like so many official statements at the time, they had the opposite effect. He recommended calm and advocated religious resignation in the face of disaster:

> I have no doubt from my investigations that there have been thousands of cases of polio here in which people got well without realising they had the disease. They had a rise in temperature, a little disturbance, a sore throat and headaches. There is no need for alarm, because that would be as if we did not believe in God's providence. This outbreak will go and it will leave little mark.[14]

I did not talk much to the other children in the ward in St Finbarr's though the beds were very close together. Dr O'Callaghan thought I was 'a typical supercilious six-year-old – you didn't mix'. This seems a little unfair. I was not used to strangers. I was frightened. Dr

O'Callaghan thought that children accepted better what was happening to them than did their parents. I found the remark annoying. It has often struck me that people – whether it be children crippled by polio in Cork in 1956 or adults during the bombing of Baghdad in 2003 – are wrongly commended by onlookers for their supposedly cheerful resignation in the face of terrifying adversity. In fact, both children and adults in such dire circumstances may only appear to accept what has happened to them because of a grim certainty on their part that there is nothing much they can do to change their fate.

Almost all those getting polio were children under the age of ten. 'None of the children cried,' said Dr O'Callaghan. 'But the worst of it was talking to the parents. They asked if their children would die or whether they would be crippled. They couldn't understand why we couldn't tell them. They were worried that their sons or daughters might get brain damage.'[15] In fact, the polio virus is highly selective in what cells it attacks. Those associated with learning are usually spared. The intelligence of the victims is not affected.

The doctors in St Finbarr's estimated that five days after the first fever became apparent – though it might have been incubating for several weeks previously – the paralysis was complete and that certainly within ten days it was as bad as it was going to get. They visited my bed once or twice a day. They would first playfully offer to shake hands. Shaking hands formally on all possible occasions has always been more common in Ireland than in England. But in this instance the purpose was to see if I could use my finger muscles. Then they would tell me to bend my knee and would ask me to try to straighten it against the pressure of their hand placed under the sole of my foot. This was to see if the muscles of the legs had weakened. They would listen to my breathing to know if the chest was being affected and ask me to bend forward to see if the muscles of the back were becoming lax.

I was vaguely aware that somewhere in the hospital, though not in my ward, there was something frightening called an 'iron lung'. I indistinctly thought of it as having monstrous qualities, the kitchen stove back at Brook Lodge come to life. There were also three 'Beavers', a version of the iron lung, which blew air into the lungs. This was too few for the number of patients who could not breathe. To keep them alive, medical students would pump air directly into their lungs through a tube in their throat, using a method that had been pioneered during a polio epidemic in Copenhagen a few years previously.

I was not the only child in the hospital who was frightened by the iron lungs. One day a thirteen-year-old girl was admitted who was having difficulty breathing. She came from an isolated part of Kerry. 'I don't think she had ever been beyond the local primary school or the church in her life,' said another patient, a twenty-six-year-old man, who saw her. 'She was put into an iron lung, which looks a bit like a high-tech coffin, but she really thought it was a coffin and made a terrible fuss. They took her out and we saw lots of medical students turning up in the ward, two every couple of hours, to keep her breathing by hand.'[16]

St Finbarr's was an old hospital with 1,200 patients on the south bank of the Lee river, but a modernised regional centre for the treatment of polio had just been established there. It treated patients from all over the south-west of

Ireland. The hospital was run by Dr Michael Goold, the Resident Medical Supervisor, a man with dark hair worn plastered down; he came from Macroom, a town west of Cork city notorious for the toughness of its inhabitants. Pauline Kent, overworked, underpaid and impatient with bureaucratic obstacles, did not like him. She thought he was 'as thick as the wall. His first priority was his job and his second was his pension. He was the pits as an administrator.' Dr O'Callaghan agrees that Goold was tough, but is more charitable. 'People were afraid of him,' she said. 'But it depended on how you handled him. He didn't like naggers.'

Dr Goold, starved of resources in an impoverished country, had been slowly renovating St Finbarr's since the end of the Second World War. But it was the nuns who were ultimately in charge of the day-to-day running of the wards. Probably medical conditions were no worse than they would have been in London or New York, but for people in Cork St Finbarr's still had the whiff of the old poorhouse it had once been, a place offering rude shelter to the destitute and the dying who had nowhere else to go. In the early 1950s most of the wards, though not the one I was in, were still heated by open fires. To reach the room where she practised physiotherapy, Pauline Kent used to walk through another room which was filled with long bundles wrapped in white hessian cloth. 'At first I thought they were filled with dirty laundry,' she said. 'Then I discovered that they contained the corpses of the very poor whose bodies had not been claimed by their relatives. They were waiting to be buried in the hospital grounds in a mass grave. There was no monument to them until one day a taxi-driver paid for a cross out of his own money.'

Andrew was in a room crowded with twenty beds – small by the standard of the hospital where there were sometimes sixty beds to a ward. All the boys were older in his ward than they were in mine, and there was a more cheerful atmosphere, though some of the children were dying. 'I had been talking to a boy who was four or five beds away. One morning I saw a nurse come and look at him and then rush out of the ward. She came back with other sisters – all nuns. I could tell by their headdresses. They held a service around the bed. Then we saw the body being wheeled away.' He was constipated – a symptom of polio in the fever stage – and constantly being given laxatives which had no effect. At first Andrew denied that he had anything more serious wrong with him than back pains, though the other boys kept telling him: 'No, you have polio like us.' Bizarrely, the only reading material was old copies of the *Field*, the glossy monthly about the agricultural activities and hobbies of the English landed classes. Andrew read an interesting article about tickling trout. He only began to understand that something was seriously wrong – and he was not just having a lucky escape from school – when after a week or more he was carried upstairs to my ward.[17] Dr O'Callaghan recalled: 'You were both very sad boys. Andrew was very much protecting you. He was trying to prevent you being lonely and used to sit on the bed chatting to you.'

With two of their sons in St Finbarr's my mother and father had taken refuge in a friendly pub in Youghal called the Wright House. It was owned by an English family of that name and, unlike Brook Lodge, it had a telephone. My father would ring up the hospital three or four times a day to ask about Andrew and me. Sometimes at 9 a.m. the nurse would say: 'They seem to be doing well.' At noon another person answering the phone in the hospital would say: 'They seem to be doing as well as can be expected.' To my parents, fearing that at any moment they might be told that either or both us were dead, this small change in emphasis seemed horribly significant. At heart they knew that the different phraseology meant nothing, but in the vacuum of information about us, my father, his tall figure crouched in the pub's telephone call-box, could not stop himself milking the words for more than he knew they were worth. He recorded later:

> To the straining ear of the enquirer the little shift of words seemed to mean that in the last three hours things had taken a terrible turn for the worse. Why else should they have used that cautious 'as well as can be expected'? I would stand at that telephone for minutes on end, making senseless conversation, repeating what was in effect the same question in a half-dozen different ways, in the futile and unreasonable hope of luring the nurse into giving out some piece of information which in reality she could not have.

My mother was consumed with guilt over her decision to return to Ireland during the epidemic. Kitty Lee, my nanny, said she thought my mother might go mad with anxiety: 'She was beside herself when the boys were in hospital.' After ten days of compulsively mulling over the few pathetic and unrevealing words from the hospital, my parents forced themselves not to discuss the news from

St Finbarr's for more than a few minutes. They played Scrabble, a game at which my mother usually defeated my father, despite his wide vocabulary, because of her more immediate practicality.

My father feared that my mother, in believing that she was entirely responsible for her sons catching polio because of her desire to return to Ireland, was in a sense unconsciously seeking to involve herself in our fate. Horrible though this sense of guilt may be, it has its advantages over seeing oneself as a passive observer, uninvolved in the trials of a loved one. My father himself, who always had great toughness and resilience in the face of disaster, borrowed an old Underwood typewriter from the owner of the pub. He distracted himself by writing humorous and satirical pieces for *Punch*. Some people said to him that it must be difficult, in such circumstances, to write articles designed to make people laugh. He explained it really did not matter what he was writing about. He compared himself to a carpenter working while waiting for news of his sick children. It really would not matter to the carpenter if he was making a kitchen table or a roulette wheel. He later wrote: 'It may even be that to be working on something as small and intricate as a short article which is designed to make people laugh is a superior therapy, requiring a maximum concentration of attention on itself, so that even the most intrusive of other cares are excluded from the mind.'[18]

The polio virus which had infected Andrew and myself is very small, only a millionth of an inch across. One authority on the disease has worked out that 17,000 such viruses could be placed on the full stop at the end of this sentence. Viewed through an electron microscope – it is invisible through an ordinary microscope – it appears even more minute than the viruses which cause HIV, yellow fever or smallpox. Its shape is peculiarly menacing. It is a round globe, divided into fifteen plates, from which sprout short truncated arms, sometimes dividing into two, which look like sinister and misshapen trees in an apple orchard whose branches have been cut back close to the ground.[19]

The polio virus has a curious and complicated lifestyle. Like other viruses it is designed for attack. It cannot multiply until it invades the right sort of living cell. Its career is inevitably that of a parasite but a highly successful one. It is a member of one of the three groups – animals, plants and viruses – to which all living things belong. Bacteria may have 5,000 to 10,000 genes but the polio virus has fewer than ten. The aim of this tiny speck of genetic material – nucleic acid with a coat of protein molecules – is to attach itself to and then penetrate an appropriate cell inside which it can reproduce. In the case of polio a prime target – destruction or serious damage of which leads to paralysis of the limbs – are certain types of nerve cells in the spinal cord which control the movements of the arms and legs. As early as 1870 a French physician, studying tissues from a patient with polio, observed that the so-called anterior horn of grey matter in the spinal cord was shrivelled. The spinal cord is not the only, or even the main, objective of the poliomyelitis virus, but it is the damage it does here which led to its name. Coined in 1880, it comes from the Greek '*polios*' meaning 'grey' and '*myelos*' which means 'marrow'. More specifically, though this was not known at the time, it is the large motor neurons in the spine, the cells which relay information to the muscles, which are under assault from the virus.

Initial hopes in the early twentieth century of finding a vaccine capable of controlling the disease were swiftly dashed. One reason for this was that there are three different types of polio virus, each with a somewhat different mode of attack and each requiring a different antibody. They are Brunhilde, Lansing and Leon, named after the people or places where they were first identified. It was the Brunhilde or Type 1, responsible for almost all epidemics, which was spreading so rapidly through Cork that summer and which I had caught. It was known to paralyse arms, legs and sometimes the ability to breathe. Type 2 was less likely to cause paralysis, but was responsible for serious epidemics of non-paralytic polio. Type 3, though uncommon, could paralyse the limbs, but was most likely to damage the bulb or stem of the brain. It was therefore sometimes called 'bulbar' polio. This made it difficult for a victim to swallow or breathe and could rapidly lead to death. The complexities of the polio virus do not end here. Aside from the three basic types of polio there are over fifty different strains of the virus which vary in their virulence and can mutate inside the body.

The difficulty of developing a vaccine in the half-century before the Cork epidemic was further complicated by prolonged misunderstanding about how people caught the disease. As late as 1935 most specialists, despite prolonged research, believed there was only one type of virus, which entered the body through the nose, spread to the lungs and then travelled to the brain and the spine through nervous tissue. All these beliefs, without exception, were shown to be false over the next twenty years.

In reality the virus enters the body through the mouth and multiplies in the tonsils at the back of the throat and in the small intestine – the alimentary tract. It then flows back into the throat mixed with saliva or is excreted as shit. Contact with either is enough to pass on the virus. It can go on being excreted for several weeks after the first infection. This makes swimming pools or sewage particularly dangerous. But within the body of the victim the journey of this tiny particle, by now numbering many millions, is not over. It enters the lymph nodes under the arms. Ten days after the first infection, though the victim may be unaware of what is happening, these can no longer contain the quantity of polio viruses. They spill into the bloodstream. This carries it to neurons in the brain and the motor neurons in the spine. Here the virus begins its work of destruction. The proteins from the virus seek to break up the neuron, destroying its ability to produce the neurochemicals which send messages to the muscles telling them to contract. The aim of this work of destruction by the virus, like a cuckoo invading another bird's nest, is to rearrange the pieces of the host neuron so it will produce the polio virus in vast quantities. When it is entirely filled with virus it explodes and the polio virus moves to attack other neurons.

By the time of the epidemic in Cork in 1956 not only had an effective vaccine been discovered in the US but a great deal was known about how the virus operated. But there was nothing the doctors in St Finbarr's or anywhere else in the world could do to impede its progress through the body once the infection had started. They could make sure the patient rested and did not walk. This was why Andrew was carried upstairs to see me in my ward. The doctors could also keep alive, at least for a time, patients who could not breathe by placing them in an iron lung.

But, if the doctors had no cure, there was a great deal the body could do to defend itself. The great American pathologist David Bodian discovered in the 1940s that even if there was only slight paralysis of a victim it was not for lack of trying by the virus. He found that, even in these milder cases, no less than 96 per cent of the motor neurons had been attacked by it. But the antibodies also had their victories. Bodian determined that for every neuron that is invaded and destroyed by the polio virus the body's immune system successfully defends another neuron. It may be damaged by the invader but it can rebuild itself so it can still send information to a muscle. The casualty rate is important here. It requires no less than 60 per cent of the motor neurons controlling a particular muscle to be destroyed before the muscle shows any sign of weakness.

The ability of the body to defend itself and the fact that some strains of polio did not paralyse explains another startling aspect of the disease. The vast majority of victims recover. Most never know that they have had polio. Only 1 or 2 per cent of those who catch it become ill. Some 98–99 per cent have only a minor infection with nausea, a sore throat, constipation, tiredness and a headache. A smaller number get a pain in the back of the neck and a smaller number still suffer from paralysis of the arms and legs or the parts of the brain controlling breathing. Dr McCarthy and other doctors in charge of trying to control the epidemic in Cork constantly repeated that most people in the city were getting the disease, without long-term ill effect, or were protected by having contracted it many years before. But nobody likes to feel that they, and above all their children, are entering a lottery in which the polio virus just might cripple or kill them, even if the chances of this happening are around fifty to one against. Nor were people in Cork or the rest of Ireland likely to be reassured by the thought that there were tens of thousands of people, unaware that they had the disease, walking the streets but capable of carrying the virus to others.

Neither my parents nor anybody else in Cork aside from a handful of doctors understood then, or even in later years, that it was impossible to stop, and difficult even to limit, the spread of the virus. Quarantine was theoretically possible but to have any effect it would have to be total. The Department of Health lacked resources but this was not the reason officials knew they could not halt the epidemic. For all their carefully phrased equivocations at the height of the epidemic, they had circulated a long memo the previous year, in 1955, cautiously pessimistic and wholly realistic in tone. It had been sent to city managers and county secretaries in charge of the local civil service, as well as to chief medical officers. It spelled out what could and could not be done in the event of an epidemic. Entitled 'Acute Anterior Poliomyelitis', it stated firmly: 'It has been established that for each paralytic case there are many other unrecognised cases. In general, the family contacts of a case of poliomyelitis are those most heavily infected with virus and in such cases they and their immediate contacts usually excrete large quantities of virus in their stools.' But the problem was the impossibility of identifying those who had non-paralytic polio and were just as dangerous, in terms of spreading the epidemic, as those who were lying in hospital. The memo blandly admitted that with so many hidden carriers 'the best means of control at our disposal will not give results that are completely satisfactory. This is due to the widespread presence of virus and to the fact that invasion by the virus is not necessarily followed by symptoms.'[20] In other words, once under way, an epidemic was unstoppable.

Three

I have no memory of realising that my legs were floppy and I could no longer walk, still less that this might be permanent. I can recollect discovering that I could no longer sit up in bed because my back muscles were weakened. Two or three pillows had to be placed under my head so I could sit in my bed to eat. The virus acts quickly. After ten days the fever had gone. The doctors needed the beds in St Finbarr's for others who had just caught polio and were pouring in from the city and the county. After three weeks, on 23 October, I was carried downstairs into an ambulance and driven a short distance north across the River Lee to a newly built orthopaedic hospital with 144 beds called St Mary's, at Gurranebraher, on a steep hill overlooking the centre of Cork.

It was a horrible place. Its single-storey isolation blocks had been built for TB patients. It had only opened the previous year and had been rapidly converted for the use of polio victims. I was lonely because Andrew had gone home. I asked if Andrew was coming with me and was told: 'No, he is going back to your house.' Soon after Andrew was first admitted to St Finbarr's a doctor or nurse had told my father that it was he who was most likely to be crippled for life. They suspected he would be unable even to sit upright. This was presumably because he had been diagnosed late, several days after me. In the event the only part of his body to suffer long-term damage was the big toe of his left foot.

The nurses in Gurranebraher maintained a gruff, bar-rack-room discipline. For food we were given thin, watery mince and badly boiled, soapy potatoes. My mother and father brought me toys, but there was an atmosphere of violence in the ward and the toys were usually broken by other boys in a few days and thrown on a rubbish heap. There was a wire attached to a single brown earphone sprouting out of the wall near each bed so patients could listen to the radio. 'The earphones were the only form of entertainment,' says Anne O'Sullivan, a nurse who had just joined the hospital. 'But they were broken in no time.'[1] They were in any case more suit-able for the adult TB patients for whom they were designed than for small children. Maureen O'Sullivan, a tireless voluntary nurse who operated a Red Cross ambu-lance, told me later, apparently struggling to find some-thing nice to say about the place, that St Mary's 'wasn't too bad. It lacked professional staff and there was a shortage of trained people. It was completely over-strained. Many of the nurses looked at it just as a job and not as a vocation. The real problem was always lack of resources.'[2] My father thought the same. He wrote that a considerable part of the everyday care of the chil-dren 'seemed to be largely in the hands of maids – young country girls with no special training at all. There were almost no arrangements for the entertainment or education of the children, who were provided with beds and expert medical attention, and nothing else.'[3]

My father's suspicion of what was wrong at the hospital was more or less exactly confirmed by an inspector from the Department of Health who visited the Cork hospitals at the end of August to see how they were coping with the epidemic. He was told by Dr O'Connell, the senior doctor at Gurranebraher, that 'the Matron was finding the recruitment of nurses very difficult, but that maids are no trouble'.[4] The shortage of nurses was partly self-inflicted. A strange aspect of nursing in Ireland at the time was that any nurse, indeed any woman working in government service, had to resign when she got married. At the height of the epidemic these married nurses were allowed to come back but they were not allowed to take permanent jobs.[5]

My bed was in the middle of the ward by a window. Once I woke up and heard a nurse telling a small boy who had messed his bed that if he did it again he would have to eat his own shit. I had difficulty sleeping after that. I was frightened that the same thing might happen to me. One night it very nearly did. I was too weak to get out of bed. I called for a bedpan, but I did not dare shout too loudly because this enraged the nurses. Nobody came. I was able to move my bottom a little and shat into a copy of the *Beano* which somebody had given me. Then I wrapped up the mess in page after page of the comic and threw it as far as I could on to the floor in the centre of the ward, but I could not see where it had landed. I spent the rest of the night and the following day in frozen terror in case the package would be discovered, opened and traced to me.

The hospital was wholly under the control of Dr St John O'Connell, a tall, strikingly good-looking man from Mallow in north Cork, who had been working for a year to make sure that its medical facilities were equivalent to anything in England. 'He was highly trained and had been in the RAF,' said Pauline Kent. 'He loved racing and used to go to all the big race meetings at York, Ascot and the Derby.'[6] Others in the hospital believed that he owned racehorses. He had returned to Ireland in 1953 and had worked briefly at St Finbarr's, where he was put in charge of two geriatric wards and conceived a low opinion of Dr Goold. Dr O'Connell's weekly round of the ward, when he came accompanied by a team of other doctors and assistants, was a regal ceremony feared by nurses and patients alike. John Creedon, an eighteen-year-old apprentice carpenter from Ballingeary, near Gougane Barra, a famous beauty spot and religious shrine in West Cork, had like me just entered Gurranebraher, badly crippled in the legs and upper body. He remembers that Dr O'Connell was 'a big, big hefty man and everybody would jump to attention when he was around. He was the king of the place.'[7] But the day-to-day running of the wards and blocks – as in other Irish hospitals at the time – was in the hands of a matron and nurses, lay rather than religious as at St Finbarr's. The nurses' chief fear was that the matron, a tall woman with a beaked nose who made sporadic night-time inspections, would catch them all playing cards. She was said to drink but her approach to our block down a concrete path was silent, and one nurse was usually on sentry duty to watch for her approach.

As more and more children disappeared into St Finbarr's

and Gurranebraher at the height of the epidemic between July and September, many in Cork suspected they were being lied to about the spread of polio and the number of its victims. 'There were rumours everywhere in the city that dead bodies were being carried out the back door of St Finbarr's at night,' said Pauline Kent, the physiotherapist who tried to revive muscles damaged by the disease. Born with an ingrained distrust of government authority stemming from their experience of foreign rule, many in Cork were firm believers in the old nostrum: 'Don't believe anything until it is officially denied.' My father shared this general scepticism about the good intentions of the authorities. It was one of the reasons he felt half at home in Ireland. 'Governments do as much harm as they can and as much good as they must,' he would say genially. Such remarks won him a reputation for cynicism but his purpose was less to condemn the state and all its works than to promote the belief that governments were far more easily influenced by individual and popular action than was generally supposed.

Belief that the authorities are lying their heads off about the number of dead and injured in any crisis is, in any case, not a uniquely Irish characteristic. In every war or disturbance I covered as a journalist from Port-au-Prince to Baghdad or Grozny, sensible people have been quite genuinely convinced that the casualty rate is far higher than anybody is admitting. They will furiously argue for the larger figure, as if to accept that the number slaughtered might have been in the hundreds rather than the thousands somehow lets the perpetrators off the hook.

In the epidemic in Cork in 1956 it was impossible to know the number of victims of polio because of the nature of the disease itself. Tens of thousands of people in this compact little city of 75,000 people – though some of the worst-affected districts were newly built suburbs just outside the city limits – were catching it without knowing or suffering long-term injuries. As early as the middle of August Dr Saunders said hopefully that the illness might be burning itself out because of a lack of new victims – everybody had already contracted it:

> He felt there was a possible reduction in the incidence in the city and suburbs now because it was accepted in an outbreak of this nature that for every case detected there were one or two hundred undetected or undiagnosed in the community, principally among children.[8]

The number of people admitted to hospital with polio is easier to discover though the official figures do not quite add up. The explanation for this is probably not very sinister, just a genuine confusion in distinguishing between those who had long-term injuries and those who had contracted polio but had since recovered. Dr O'Callaghan says that 546 patients had passed through St Finbarr's by the end of the epidemic early in 1957, which is probably accurate enough.[9] This suggests, going by Dr Saunders's figure (borne out by polio specialists in other parts of the world) for the relationship between cases diagnosed and cases undetected, that at least 50,000 people caught polio in Cork city and county over this period. A further source of confusion is that health officials, city politicians, local business and the newspapers in Cork were overeager – seeing their shops empty and themselves treated as pariahs – to claim the epidemic had largely ended earlier than it had. There is little about it in the papers after the middle of September, though I myself only entered St Finbarr's on 30 September. Dr O'Callaghan says the epidemic continued at slower pace, with only a couple of admissions a week, well into the following year: 'The peak was in August and September, but they kept coming into early 1957 with the last patients arriving in March and April.'

There was a suspicion in Cork that the epidemic had spread to Dublin and people were dying like flies in its fever hospitals after being intentionally misdiagnosed as suffering from other diseases. They believed, so my father later recorded, that 'due to the savage wiles and intrigues of the Dubliners, the newspapers had been, as the Irish saying goes, "brought to see" that it would not be in their interests to report the state of affairs in Dublin. Instead they should concentrate on ruining poor Cork.' In private the health officials in Dublin were indeed worried that the epidemic might spread northwards and they carefully watched the number of admissions to hospitals in the capital, but there is no evidence that they concealed outbreaks of polio. By 21 July, just as the epidemic was raging in Cork, there had been only twelve cases in Dublin over the previous seven months.[10] Suspicions were also voiced that small towns, for base commercial reasons, were keeping quiet about polio. Irish towns and villages often have a dim view of each other. A correspondent writing to the Department of Health claimed that 'in Youghal a woman got polio and it was hushed [up] apparently, so we heard, to avoid ruining this seaside resort – just for a season. What about the young lives that could

51

be ruined for life?'[11] The story about Youghal was certainly untrue. So far from keeping quiet about polio in the town, the nuns at the Loreto convent where Andrew and I had gone to school, closed down the school for three days in October so staff and pupils could pray for our recovery.

The one place where information about the epidemic was demonstrably suppressed was in Cork city itself. From the beginning the *Cork Examiner* and the *Evening Echo*, powerful organs in this small community, had reported the epidemic accurately but gingerly, never dwelling on its devastating impact on the economic life of the city. Their attitude was very important because the *Cork Examiner* in particular was an excellent paper, crucial in shaping local opinion. Polio stories were almost always on the front page but never as the lead story. The headline would give the dire news about the number of new victims, but the sub-headline was almost always upbeat, invariably citing some local authority as claiming there was 'No Occasion for Undue Alarm', 'Outbreak Not Yet Dangerous Says Doctor' and 'Panic Reaction Without Justification'. Even after half a century this constant drumbeat of bogus reassurance has exactly the opposite impact than the one intended, giving an impression not of confidence but of half-suppressed panic. There are no reports, for instance, of the mass exodus of children from better-off families to stay with relatives elsewhere in the country, though Alan Crosbie, later the chief executive of the *Cork Examiner*, was evacuated as a child to Dublin to stay with his grandmother for a year and so avoid the epidemic.

There was a further reason why the newspapers played down polio in Cork. My father always told me that the newspapers had been leaned on by businesses in Cork to conceal the extent of the epidemic. He claimed that 'the owners of some of the biggest stores in the city made a démarche. In deputation to the newspapers they threatened to withdraw advertising from such newspapers as might continue to report regularly and in detail on the polio epidemic.' I wondered in later years if this was true, since rumours that newspapers are being leaned on by their advertisers are common and usually false (in part because newspapers know in advance what will offend their advertisers so no pressure is necessary). But reading old copies of the *Cork Examiner* from 1956 it is noticeable that after 12 September references to polio abruptly slow to a trickle. This may partially reflect the facts. There were fewer victims as the month went on. But the epidemic was certainly not over. I remember other admissions after I entered St Finbarr's at the end of September. Even a fall in the number of new cases does not quite explain the sudden cessation of the previous bland but frequent and detailed reports.

A file in the Department of Health archives, unnoticed for half a century, is evidence that my father was right in believing that the big retail advertisers in Cork did not want to hear any more about the epidemic and had taken steps to ensure that nobody else heard about it either. Hoteliers in the city had been badly hit. An article in *The Times* of London said they had lost 75 per cent of their customers.[12] The Irish Tourist Association had a simple solution to the problems of businesses in Cork whose customers had disappeared, staying out of the city and the county because they were understandably frightened of catching polio. It noted that:

> The publicity given by the newspapers to the incidence of polio in Cork was injudicious, in as much as it had the effect of creating a scary atmosphere, and was thus a contributory if not the sole cause of the reportedly heavy trading losses suffered by hoteliers and the business community in the area during this year's tourist season.

All would be well, it said, if the Department of Health simply treated as confidential all information about patients suffering from infectious diseases in the hospitals. One official was appalled by the idea and indignantly minuted on the proposal:

> I for one would feel very annoyed if I came to Cork on a holiday with my family and found polio raging and that the business people were prepared to allow me to come and to expose my family to the disease – for the sake of my money as a tourist.

He thought the public had the right to know everything about any infectious diseases they might catch. But another official, confirming my father's account, wrote that 'the real fault lies with the press and I know the *Cork Examiner* has been taken to task by the business community of Cork'.[13]

As the epidemic entered its third month it had become well known in Britain despite the efforts of health officials in Cork to play it down. Some 250 dockers in Liverpool went on strike on 27 August after they were asked to unload a ship called the *Glengariff* on which a seaman, diagnosed shortly after arrival as having polio, had travelled from Cork. The strikers said they were refusing to work until the ship was certified as safe. 'All we want to do is safeguard our families.' Dockers working on two other ships in Liverpool went on sympathy strike. The *Glengariff*, a coaster, was isolated in a far corner of the Liverpool docks to reassure the men. Rather less reassuring were the words of Dr J. B. Meredith, the Liverpool Deputy Medical Officer, who said: 'I think there is no more risk in working the ship than in dealing with any other coming from ports where polio may be present.'[14]

The *Glengariff* had in fact arrived in Liverpool more than three weeks earlier on 4 August, but it was only a few days later that one of the passengers, Raymond Smith, a nineteen-year-old seaman originally from Liverpool, was discovered to have polio. BBC radio broadcast an SOS message before the main news bulletin on 8 August asking thirty-one saloon passengers, whose names were unknown and might have been infected by Smith, to report immediately to a doctor.[15] The announcement had presumably alerted the dockers to the possible dangers involved when it came to unloading the ship some three weeks later. Dr Jack Saunders, the Medical Officer of Health in Cork, later wrote a stern letter to the *British Medical Journal* and the *Lancet* claiming that Smith must have contracted polio in Glasgow. It is a measure of how many people with polio were misdiagnosed that a doctor in Scotland had told Smith that he had laryngitis and another doctor in Cork that he was suffering from a slipped disc. Dr

Saunders said the young seaman was only in Cork for a few days before sailing for Liverpool and 'the incubation [for polio] is about twelve days'. Smith must therefore have been infected before he arrived. Saunders went on to criticise 'the exaggerated newspaper notoriety afforded to the poliomyelitis epidemic in Cork'. He accepted, but in rather a regretful tone, that the BBC had done the right thing in publicising the polio case on board the *Glengariff*.[16]

The self-defeating tendency of health officials and local politicians in Cork to minimise the impact of polio was little different from the response of their counterparts in other parts of the world when faced with an epidemic or any other disaster. During crises in any country a common feature is often a tirade by the authorities against popular panic, usually an unintentional sign of the officials' own anxiety. There is also nothing out of the ordinary in official dislike of the press and publicity, frequently blamed for exaggerating the scale of the problem. But in the Cork epidemic there was an extra element, an exaggerated sensitivity to any criticism emanating from Britain. Thirty-five years after the British withdrawal, Irish self-confidence was still very brittle. In September a British Sunday newspaper published an article describing Cork as a 'city in panic'. This provoked an outburst of hysterical rage on the part of the local councillors. Sean Casey, the Lord Mayor of Cork, said the report was beneath contempt, adding: 'Press publicity, which is ill-advised and ill-informed, has done immeasurable damage to the traders of the city.' An irate councillor played the patriotic card, claiming: 'Cross-channel Sunday newspapers were not slow to publish anything which tended to discredit the Irish people.'[17] He said such papers should be boycotted. Business and patriotic opinion had reached the same conclusion. By the time I was being taken by ambulance to St Finbarr's, a reader of the local papers in Cork would have concluded that the epidemic was finished.

I was in Gurranebraher for thirteen weeks. I could sometimes move about the ward on crutches and with my legs in steel callipers, struts of metal on either side of the leg with pieces of leather to keep the limb rigid. My back was supported by a hard plastic waistcoat like a corset. Mostly, however, when I left my bed at all, I was in a wheelchair. My parents would visit twice a week. Kitty Lee took the bus from Youghal thirty miles away, got off below Guarranebraher hill and then walked up to the hospital. 'I brought you comics and books,' she said. 'We found a small place where we could read. The nurses seemed nice to me.'[18] In fact, this meant that she would read to me, since I was only just beginning to spell out words.

My father had noticed that the nurses were ill-trained and inconsiderate. But he was prone, particularly in Ireland, to find economic reasons for the failings and ill behaviour of others. He believed that most of the patients came from miserably poor families. This was not entirely true, since polio was at its worst in the newly built and relatively well-off southern suburbs of Cork. Maureen O'Sullivan, the voluntary nurse from the Red Cross, mostly picked up patients who 'came front affluent areas in the city; they were often well-nourished, well-cared-for children'. But no doubt some of the patients were very poor. At that time in Ireland this meant they had nothing at all or at best a small farm. In the slums of north Cork the houses were mainly filled with women since many of the men were working on building sites in England repairing bomb damage. My father wrote: 'I met one mother who lived in the far west of County Cork and was able to visit her paralysed son only once in four months – on the day that there was a big football match in Cork city and the railway ran a very cheap day excursion from her village.'

My mother was equally appalled. 'The children were merely regarded as things to be washed, fed and doctored. It was nobody's fault. The epidemic had overwhelmed the health services. The hospital was reminiscent of the Crimean War, with beds nearly touching and some children lying on mattresses on the floor.'[19]

Not all the children were unhappy. The older ones were quicker to adapt and less vulnerable. John Creedon, after spending three weeks in St Finbarr's at about the same time as myself, had been moved to another block where the patients were older. He did not find the food bad but added wryly: 'the food wasn't much better at home'. He and other young men from the country would walk out of the hospital to farms just beyond its northern boundary. 'We liked to see the farmers sowing because we came from farms ourselves.'[20]

Other boys teased me because I was Anglo-Irish and spoke with an English accent. I was not yet old enough to have given much thought to the problems of national identity. I knew I was not English. I remembered Kitty's warnings about them. But I also knew that I was not exactly Irish either. My father had once tried to explain our family's complicated ethnic origins by telling me I had Scottish blood. I was none too sure who or what Scotland was but I unwisely passed this on to other boys in the ward. They began to shout 'Scottish Bloodman! Scottish Bloodman!' whenever they saw me.

I became completely silent and refused to talk to anybody. The doctors, always seeking a physical explanation for any ailment, believed that the virus might have damaged the muscles controlling my vocal cords. My father could see that my physical condition was slightly improving. The callipers allowed me to move a few tottering steps with the use of long wooden crutches under my armpits, and the corset-like plastic waistcoat supported my back, though it was sweaty in hot weather and the bottom of the plastic rubbed against my hips. But at the same time my father noticed that 'he who had been so gay, so alert, inquisitive and talkative seemed to be sinking into a voiceless apathy'. A few weeks later I would only speak in a whisper. I have little real memory of this though I recall a soothing sense of withdrawal from the world around me. The nurses and other patients, who both made me feel acutely vulnerable, became a more distant presence. My parents decided, probably rightly, that I was dying.

My parents asked the doctors if there was any essential medical reason why I should stay in Gurranebraher. After two or three weeks' delay, deeply frustrating for my parents who could see me fading away before their eyes, the doctors said I could go home and I returned to Brook Lodge. Once there I began to recover my spirits. Most of the time I could only crawl because my legs were so weak, but my arms were unaffected and soon became unnaturally strong. My mother was good at finding things which I could do despite my injuries. My legs, particularly my right leg, were shrunken and too weak to support my weight. I still wore the plastic waistcoat. It was unclear when the muscles on both sides of my back would be strong enough for me to sit up unsupported without distorting the shape of my spine. Kitty would carry me on her back to the bottom of the front field where I would sit on a grassy bank amid the rabbit burrows and pick primroses. I could operate close to the floor without difficulty. I painted all the skirting boards in my nursery a slightly bilious green, which I could do lying on my stomach. I needed to be carried downstairs and then placed in a wheelchair with a green canvas back. I learned to read and play chess.

A year later I went to Whitechapel hospital in London for a series of operations on my feet, the purpose of which was to transfer the muscles, which had survived, to do the work of those that had died. After a few years I gave up the callipers and the waistcoat and I finally discarded the crutches when I was ten. By then polio was being rapidly eradicated. In the US the Salk vaccine had been shown to be a success. It was first used in Cork in 1957 when a small quantity of the vaccine was obtained from Canada. The Department of Health estimated in the spring of 1957 that they had just enough vaccine to protect 'children over twelve months and under three years'. It had worked out that there were about four thousand such children in Cork city.[21]

In a final nasty little twist to the epidemic, some of the precious vaccine was diverted. A few months later, as he prepared a wider vaccination programme at the end of 1957, the Health Minister denounced those in Cork who had supplied some of the vaccine to those who were ineligible to receive it: 'as a consequence some children in the groups at greatest risk were deprived of this valuable protection'.[22] In the second half of 1958 there was mass vaccination against polio for the first time in Ireland. By the early sixties polio had disappeared as an epidemic disease in the US and Western Europe.

The fear outlasted the epidemic for several years. Ted Tanner from Bandon in West Cork recalls that a year after he was released from hospital, walking on crutches and with callipers on his legs, older people would keep away from him in case he should give them the disease.[23] Maureen O'Sullivan, the Red Cross nurse, who arranged physical training for victims in the late fifties, remembers that 'at the sight of my ambulance in their street people would think that the polio was back. They would run into their houses and a few would get down on their knees to pray. They had lost all hope – they were that frightened.'[24]

As the polio virus retreated in the late 1950s under the impact of vaccination it could still inflict terrible injuries. These explain why the illness provoked such terror. In the spring of 1958 Jim Costello, an able and intelligent man who later became chairman of the Post Polio Support Group in Ireland, contracted acute respiratory poliomyelitis after attending a football match when he was fifteen years old and at school in Dublin. Almost half a century later he still has no use of his arms or hands, is paralysed in his upper body and has severe breathing difficulties. He spent six years in different hospitals in

Ireland and England. To breathe at all he needs an 'iron lung ventilator' for fourteen to sixteen hours a day during the three to four days a week he spends in hospital, and a ventilator with a nose fitting when he is at home. He has a brace to support his spine and a special machine called 'Distaff' to sign his name, a device invented during the Second World War for people whose arms had been amputated.[25]

Even for a generation which has no personal experience of polio the disease is still remembered with dread. In a bizarre illustration of this, President George W. Bush was accused in 2001 of describing the famed rapper Eminem as 'the most dangerous threat to American children since polio'. Publicity posters for the music star carrying these distasteful words were plastered on walls across the US and Britain. It may be that the quote was fabricated in order either to publicise Eminem or to discredit George Bush, but its use shows that polio is still perceived as the epitome of evil.

Four

In the weeks before the epidemic I had been building a tree house fifty yards from the front of Brook Lodge with pieces of an old door and a tea chest in a giant lime tree overlooking the road to Youghal. Sitting in my tree house, hidden by the pale green leaves, I liked to look at people, unaware that they were being observed, travelling below on bicycles or in horse-drawn carts and ageing cars. Charlie the dog also enjoyed the place because between the bottom of the tree and the road there was a high stone wall with a hole in it where several large stones had fallen out. Through the hole, its position masked by the long grass, he could bark furiously at dogs passing on the road without fear of retaliation.

I had another, slightly more dangerous tree house built using a discarded light blue child's playpen in a tall sycamore at the back of the house, from which I could see the kitchen yard, the walled garden and, across the roof of a shed, the courtyard where the gig and trap were left when not taking us to Youghal. The branches of the tree hung over the ruins of an outbuilding of which the roof had long rotted away and which was used as a rubbish dump. Pink flowers and damp green moss grew in the crevices in its walls. It was inhabited mainly by cats rummaging for food among the garbage and hopeful of finding a rat, though these were in short supply because they were the only animals of which my mother was truly frightened. To keep them at bay she fed a tribe of fifteen cats, though only five of them were allowed to enter the house, a right they defended with ferocious enthusiasm against the cats who lived in the yard outside the kitchen and in the walled garden.

It had been a bad moment for the rat population in Brook Lodge when my mother and father took it over after retreating to Ireland in 1947. The house was derelict. The Reverend Drew, who built the beautiful Georgian part of the building, and his descendants had long departed to their neo-Gothic stronghold at Heathfield Towers, leaving empty plinths where once had stood the two stone lions. The house fell into decay over the years. My mother Patricia had discovered it, engulfed by overgrown shrubs and brambles, when out riding. On seeing it Olive Arbuthnot, my grandmother, protested in vain against her daughter living there. She said: 'You can't live in that dump, it's worse than a ruined Norman keep.'

The only inhabitant was an old man who lived in one room where the ceiling had not fallen in. He wore a ragged black cutaway coat and sat on a chair beneath an enormous crucifix reading sacred books in Latin. The rest of the downstairs rooms were inhabited by chickens, the occasional cow and, so my mother reported with alarm, 'about 20,000 rats'. These soon made their presence felt during the initial phase of reconstruction. Almost all the glass in the five enormous windows on the ground floor was broken. One of the few panes to survive was in the window of the dining room where somebody had cut into the glass with diamond the words 'Christmas 1856'. Patricia first replaced the glass in the windows of the drawing room. By the following morning all the newly installed panes had fallen out and were lying broken on the ground. Overnight hordes of rats had eaten all the fresh putty. She then mixed rat poison with the next batch of putty and the glass stayed in. For a more permanent solution to the rat problem she imported those cats.

The house had no electricity, no sewerage, and water had to be pumped by hand from a deep well. On the other hand it cost only 120 pounds a year under a thirty-three-year lease. Workers were available in Youghal, a town sunk deep in depression, for very little money. A slight hiccup here was that the old man who owned the house had died just after he concluded negotiations on the lease, and some said his ghost haunted the corridors of Brook Lodge, giving pause to those seeking employment there. My father sought to persuade potential employees that the ghost had been a man of great good will when alive and there was no reason to suppose that his character had deteriorated now that he was dead. He said his sensible argument failed to quell their fears, but ultimately a number of workers were persuaded to carry out sufficient repairs to make the house habitable.

My parents had very little money. Although my mother's family was rich, she had been cut off when she left her first husband and took up with my father in 1939. Friendly relations were restored but her allowance only amounted to two to three hundred pounds a year. A local firm, asked to provide an estimate for installing plumbing, demanded five hundred pounds for construction of the cesspit alone. My mother, always confident of her ability to solve practical problems, decided she would have to build it herself. She went to the sanitary inspector in Cork and asked him how to make a cesspit. He was surprised but made some rough drawings. She hired two local gravediggers for fifteen pounds who dug busily in a corner of the walled garden and had soon excavated a deep pit. When it was covered over, the sanitary inspector, who had to give permission for its use, came to Brook Lodge, proclaimed it the finest cesspit he had ever seen and took my mother and the gravediggers off to the pub for a celebratory drink.

The gravediggers had been easy to hire because in those gloomy post-war years Youghal and the rest of Ireland was sliding into ever deeper decay. One day a man organising the delivery of construction materials to Brook Lodge drew my father aside and whispered that he could offer a significant discount on his price. His one condition was that the bricks and cement had to be delivered between three and five in the morning. He explained that the lorries delivering the materials had to cross the Blackwater from County Waterford to reach us in County Cork. The long iron bridge which spanned the river just above Youghal was visibly rusting away. Fishermen sailing beneath it in their small boats, who glanced up at the rotting structure above their heads, nervously reported that they would never travel over it again. Local engineers insisted that rows of barrels filled with cement and with a plank across the top be placed at regular intervals on the bridge, forcing drivers to weave in and out, thereby reducing their speed to five miles an hour. Heavy trucks, blamed for much of the damage, were banned at all times.

They were compelled to cross the Blackwater over a safer bridge ten miles further north upriver at Cappoquin making a round trip of twenty miles over a slow winding road. Watchmen were supposed to enforce strictly the new regulations. But at night these men either went home, fell asleep or were paid off by the truck drivers who drove across the bridge, negotiating their way with difficulty around the speed barriers, delivered their loads to the other side of the river and then whisked back to County Waterford before dawn.

I am suspicious of my memories of Brook Lodge before I was taken to hospital. Given what was about to happen to me, it is not surprising that everything to do with the house is suffused with a golden glow of warmth and happiness. It is also true that memoirs of the Anglo-Irish gentry frequently begin with a lyrical account of childhood spent in a decaying country house in the midst of the lush Irish countryside. Autobiographies by Roman Catholic Irish are traditionally more dour affairs, describing an early youth passed amid poverty, disease and savage beatings by their schoolteachers. But in my case I was very happy growing up in Brook Lodge. It had everything a child could want – aside perhaps from other children, but I did not feel this as much of a loss. There were streams to dam, trees to climb and animals to be observed in the stables and the fields. Behind a screen in the older part of the house were boxes full of old military uniforms covered in gold braid in which to dress up. I was always protected by Kitty Lee so I was not as vulnerable as other boys of my age to the small setbacks and rebuffs of childhood.

I do not think I was more than vaguely conscious of my parents' lack of money, though this could explain why I was so obsessed with filling my money box. In later years I would find that my father had endlessly scribbled worried little financial calculations on the endpapers of books he was reading. The outgoings always seemed greater than the income from freelance articles he had succeeded in selling. I certainly did not know about writs being served for the non-payment of bills. In any case, by the time I was of an age to be even dimly conscious of such things my father was having increasing success as a writer and journalist, though he still had to operate under a bewildering number of noms de plume. He told in his memoirs how a guest at Brook Lodge had described the strange 'literary colony' which inhabited it. In reality the only writer in the place was my father, working under different names:

He claimed to have met Frank Pitcairn, ex-correspondent of the *Daily Worker* – a grouchy, disillusioned type secretly itching to dash out and describe a barricade. There was Claud Cockburn, talkative, boastful of past achievements and apt, at the drop of a hat, to tell, at length, the inside story of some forgotten diplomatic crisis of the 1930s. Patrick Cork would look in – a brash little number and something of a professional Irishman, seeking, no doubt, to live up to his name. James Helvick lived in and on the establishment, claiming that he needed quiet with plenty of good food and drink to enable him to finish a play and a novel which would soon bring enough money to repay all costs. In the background, despised by the others as a mere commercial hack, Kenneth Drew hammered away at the articles which supplied the necessities of the colony's life.[1]

By the time I was five or six my parents were not as flat broke as they had been at the time I was born. My grandfather Jack Arbuthnot, who died in 1950, had not cut my mother out of his will as he had threatened when she left her first husband Arthur Byron in 1939, but the income from his estate went to my grandmother Olive Arbuthnot until her death in 1953. At the time I went to St Finbarr's my father was working successfully for *Punch*, and two different collections of stories he had written for the magazine would soon be published. John Huston had recently filmed *Beat the Devil*. The first volume of his autobiography *In Time of Trouble* came out to acclaim from reviewers in 1956 and was rapidly reprinted. He found his conventional and gentlemanly publisher Rupert Hart-Davis pleased that the book was a success, but a little dismayed that it was written by such a notorious radical.

It was not just in contrast to an Irish fever hospital, or through the mists of Anglo-Irish nostalgia, that Brook Lodge appeared an enchanting house. Light streamed into its high and graceful Georgian rooms through the great windows. Wherever you stood or sat inside you looked out on the luxuriant greens of the Irish countryside. Around the house were lawns, covered in daffodils and tulips in spring, and beyond, a circle of tall dark green yew trees. Far away across the fields were the wooded hills at the mouth of the Blackwater valley and a silver streak where the river broadened out as it reached the estuary. But the beauty of the landscape was not the only, or even the main, attractive feature of Brook Lodge. The house owed its vigorous personality to our lack of money, which ensured that it never saw the hand of a contractor and was reconstructed piecemeal by my mother.

The entrance to Brook Lodge was through black iron gates in a semicircular plastered stone wall, which appeared abruptly on the right side of the narrow road from Youghal. Celandines, their delicate yellow flowers open in daytime and closed in the fading evening light, grew in the soft wet earth of the verge. Visitors often missed the turn and drove past it, disappearing into a tangle of muddy boreens, steep hills and little valleys. A short drive with grass down the middle led from the gate past the yew trees to the front of the house. The large double doors, in the centre of each of which was a round inlaid brass door knocker with a ring in the mouth of a lion, opened into a cavernous and dimly lit hall. On the wall by the doors hung a picture of a dark-featured man with a pointed beard, black hat and lowering expression whom I imagined to be Guy Fawkes. Smiling across at him, from the other side of the hall, was a picture in an ornate frame of a French court lady, simpering and heavily rouged, in a low-cut ball dress.

There was a grey marble fireplace, but it was never lit except at Christmas when a Christmas tree was erected at the far end of the hall. Cats often huddled against the wall beside the fireplace, absorbing heat from the the drawing-room fire burning on the other side of the wall. The drawing room, my father's study and the dining room were entered directly from the hall. At the far end was an elegant staircase with rickety banisters leading to the upper storey where there was the nursery and the bedrooms of my parents, Andrew and myself. There was also a semicircular room, used as a boxroom, the ceiling of which had fallen in long before. In one corner was a ladder and if you climbed it, then walked along a beam, you could reach the trapdoor which led to the roof. Whenever the drip coming through the ceiling of my bedroom turned into a torrent Paddy McMahon would disappear up the ladder carrying a bucket of hot tar to mend holes in the lead.

It was never a convenient building. The architect, determined on classical proportions, had devoted an inordinate amount of space to halls and corridors. He assumed that there would be numerous servants to make up fires in every room. Steps led into the older house, with low ceilings and rough wooden beams, to which it was attached at one corner. Here it was easy to see what Olive Arbuthnot had meant about Brook Lodge looking like a ruined Norman keep. On the ground floor there was the harness room, smelling of polished leather, with saddles resting on a pointed wooden rack and harness hanging from the walls. Beside it was the room used as the larder, though it was seldom cooler than any other room in the house, its door always closed against marauding cats. Next door was another room where coal, anthracite and turf were stored. In the corridor immediately outside this was a shallow pool of water. The electric pump, which had replaced an outdoor handpump for drawing water from the deep well in the courtyard, constantly dripped. The pump worked well for about thirty years, but the leak persisted despite all efforts to mend it. I enjoyed splashing through it when riding my tricycle. Once past the puddle you were in the kitchen, reasonably well heated by an Aga and a stove for heating the water. On the floor above was Paddy's room, which we were never allowed to enter, the bathroom and my oldest brother Alexander's bedroom, which had a beehive in a disused chimney in the thick outer wall. The bees counter-attacked briskly and effectively when anyone tried to dislodge them.

As a small child, not very tall for my age, I became very familiar with pieces of furniture which were my height. In the centre of the drawing room I was fascinated by a little round Regency mosaic table, which came up to my chest, and had a circular pattern of red-and-yellow flowers and green leaves inlaid in a black stone background. I used to draw my finger along a little ragged fissure, a line of missing stones ripped from the table's surface by the blast from the V-1 rocket which blew up my parents' house in St John's Wood in 1944. (My brother Andrew many years later met a German rocket scientist called Dieter Schwebs, then resident in Washington and a former employee of the Pentagon, who had helped design the guidance system of the V-1. Andrew mentioned to him the destruction of our St John's Wood house. 'Good heffens!' exclaimed the scientist in dismay, startled at meeting a member of a family which had been victims of his handiwork. 'Nobody hurt. I trust.'

There were as many horses as people at Brook Lodge. The stables and a barn for storing hay were in a long one-storey building, made out of cement blocks with a corrugated-iron roof, to the right of the house. My mother was seeking to relieve our penury by selling ponies, bought from tinkers, now called Travellers, many of whom were recognisable by their bright red hair. (In times of need the tinkers sometimes bought broken antique furniture from us which they would repair and sell.) She also bred weight-carrying hunters. I was told to keep out of one of the stables which contained an ill-tempered but valuable mare called Sheila. She once tried to kill Patricia by lashing out at her with her hoofs when she was crossing a field. Fortunately for my mother the hoof hit a bucket she was carrying, but even so its metal rim was driven deep into her leg, forcing her to lie in bed for six weeks. In her stable Sheila had to be satisfied with smaller prey. I would listen for the crash of her hoof when, after trapping a rat in the corner of her stable, she would wait for it to make a dart for safety and stamp it to death.

At the age of three I was allowed to ride around on a white donkey called Jacky, sitting in a comfortable basketwork saddle strapped to his back, like an Indian howdah on a miniature elephant. Later Paddy McMahon would take me in a gig to the Loreto convent, on a bluff close to a white-painted lighthouse at the far end of Youghal overlooking the mouth of the Blackwater. The horse used for the school trip was Blackie, whose only bad habit was a fondness for ice cream. On seeing a child with an ice-cream cone standing on the pavement after coming out of Paisley's, the main grocer in town, she would turn her head and scoop up the ice cream with her large tongue.

My mother had ridden everywhere as a girl, both to go fox-hunting and to visit her friends. The Anglo-Irish landowners had hunted for centuries, the event being conducted along the lines of a cavalry charge, with the horses surging over the high Irish banks and stone walls.

After the loss of their lands because of the land acts and the end of their remaining political influence at the time of Irish independence in 1921, hunting became an obsession, central to their social life and sense of identity. Hunting in England was considered anaemic and regarded with some contempt. Casualties among the riders were often heavy and this was seen as inevitable. My mother rode very well, normally with the West Waterford pack, but even so she had sometimes broken bones. Once during the Boxing Day meet at Clashmore, a village filled with pubs on the other side of the Blackwater, her horse had fallen and she had been taken to the Bon Secours hospital in Cork. It was a bad day to be admitted. All the doctors were at a race meeting and she was looked after by an inexperienced nun. When my mother, her jaw clenched, began to swallow her tongue and choke, the nun panicked and, in an effort to reach the tongue, knocked out all of my mother's front teeth, compelling her to wear false teeth ever afterwards.

My brother Alexander also hunted enthusiastically, though in 1958 at the age of seventeen he suddenly appeared on television in Britain to denounce the sport as unspeakably cruel to foxes. He had gone to a television studio in support of his girlfriend Linden Zilliacus, daughter of a left-wing Labour MP. Linden was to represent the anti-hunting case in opposition to a local Master of Foxhounds. At the last moment the TV producer discovered that she did not know one end of a horse from another and asked Alexander to appear instead. He pointed out that he was pro-hunting, but the need to bail out Linden compelled him temporarily to become an apostate. Opponents of hunting watching the show were at first cheered at finding that their advocate was a fox-hunter who, sickened by his former bestial activities, had finally seen the light. But, watching him in action on the screen, they were alarmed to discover that his opposition to hunting had an original twist. After running through the standard arguments about the miserable fate of the fox, he began to denounce hunting in England as too tame: the riders timid, the horses overbred, the fences low and too easily jumped. He compared it adversely to hunting in Ireland where the riders were in almost as much danger as the foxes. He had hoped that our mother would not hear of his temporary anti-hunting posture, but of course news spread rapidly via stunned relatives and within forty-eight hours he was having to explain to Patricia the reasons behind his apparent treachery.

I had no idea about my father's political notoriety until I began to suspect at about the age of ten that we were not a typical Anglo-Irish family. His communist past never had much impact in Youghal, though there were suspicions that he was an active Freemason. These were fed by the frequent visits to Brook Lodge of the local Protestant sexton, an undoubted Freemason who in reality was there because of his second and part-time job which was to serve summonses for the non-payment of bills. This caused less comment than in Britain or the US. Being hounded by bailiffs has always elicited more popular sympathy in Ireland, with its long memory of evictions for non-payment of rent, than in England.

I was a frequent visitor to Claud's study on the ground floor, a long room, unique in Brook Lodge because at one end it had a double-glazed window and was therefore kept pleasantly warm by a single electric heater. Nobody was allowed to tidy it. The floor, the sofa and the chairs were all covered with crumpled newspapers, books, sheets of carbon paper and discarded typescripts. My father sat before his typewriter at his desk by the window or in a dark red leather armchair. There was always a Woodbine cigarette in his long tapering fingers stained brown from nicotine and black with ink from carbon papers. It is a measure of his tolerance that he showed no resentment at my frequent visits because the reason for them cannot have been entirely to his liking. To supplement the cash in my black money box I was collecting silver paper from inside cigarette packets which, when enough was accumulated, could be sold back to a local shop. This was harmless enough except that sometimes, frustrated by finding a packet with one or two cigarettes in it I would take it away anyway. I was also on the lookout for empty pint bottles of Paddy Irish whiskey which my father had covertly brought back from Youghal in order to take a reviving nip to aid composition. These were also worth a couple of pennies each if returned to a pub and I would often remove them even if a generous measure remained at the bottom of the bottle.

Did I realise how much my father drank? When I was a young teenager I was embarrassed when he was visibly tight or fell over, all the more so because I was conscious that I was also unsteady on my legs because of polio. By then it did not take very much to make him drunk, which may have saved his life. He was always very benign however much whiskey he consumed. 'My legs refuse their function,' he would say in a surprised but amiable tone when unable to get out of his chair. 'Your father was a scream but he drank too much,' said Dick Cunningham, a farmer living near Brook Lodge, who several times helped my father home after he had fallen off his bicycle on his way back from Youghal.[2]

I spent much of my time in the walled garden which was surrounded by high stone walls. I used to watch Paddy McMahon, a tiny but vigorous old man, digging in the garden and herding the sheep. I was told he was about one hundred years old, but then lots of other people, including Kitty Lee, who was forty-three at the time, also told me they were a hundred. But in Paddy's case it was very nearly true. He had been born in 1860, a dozen years after the Great Famine, on the coast of County Clare where his family herded sheep. His father had told him how during the Famine starving potato farmers from inland had arrived on the coast looking for food. 'There wasn't a nettle in the churchyard nor a winkle on the rocks left after them, and they died on those rocks,' he said without much sympathy. At the age of eighteen, speaking little English, Paddy had gone with two cousins, who spoke only Irish, to find work in Liverpool. They arrived in a large city where their small bundles of clothes were immediately stolen, a loss which didn't surprise them since they expected little better from the English. Several weeks passed before they discovered that the city they were in was in fact Dublin. Paddy eventually found his way to Liverpool where he worked for eighteen miserable years in the docks before returning to Ireland and becoming a shepherd.

I did not see much of my brothers, Alexander and Andrew. Alexander was nine years older than me – at that age an unbridgeable gap – and since 1950, the year I was born, he had been at boarding school, first in England and then in Scotland. His absence had one advantage for me because I could bounce up and down on his bed, which had stronger springs than my own, in his room in the old part of the house. It was a low room on the second floor with wooden beams just below the flat roof, and when not jumping up and down, I would lie on the bed listening to the rain falling on the flat roof overhead. In the harness room below, where saddles and bridles were stored, Alexander kept a ferocious white ferret with red eyes called Bun with which he caught rabbits. I was frightened of Bun and kept away from the old tea chest where he lived. Alexander was by this time at Glenalmond, a public school housed in a dark pink sandstone fortress close to the Highland line outside Perth. He had returned there several weeks before Andrew and I were taken to St Finbarr's; after we had been diagnosed with polio, the school authorities remained apparently unaware, or were careful to conceal, that he too might have been infected by the virus which, on occasion, may not show symptoms for up to a month.

At the age of six my picture of the outside world, away from Brook Lodge and Youghal, was seen largely through the prism of my father's anecdotes. He told them with great verve, often talking in short bursts of words like Mr Jingle in *Pickwick Papers*. He illustrated points with rapid hand movements. The stories, often about our neighbours, were more vivid and real in my mind than my own vague observations. For instance, few of the Anglo-Irish gentry, generally little interested in politics since the overthrow of their class at the time of the British withdrawal, were much dismayed by my father's communist past. But east of Cappoquin the owner of a large mansion, supposedly once connected to MI5 or MI6, was vociferous in his denunciations. My father said he had difficulty talking to the man, not because of his fervent anti-communism, but because of his appalling bad breath. He said he suspected that a toad might have died in the man's throat, thus explaining the penetrating stench. The neighbour became known in the family as 'Toad-in-the-Throat'. I had hardly been aware of his existence before, but after listening to my father I would stare at the man's mouth hoping to see a sign of the dead toad.

Visitors to Brook Lodge were few. Aunt Joan, my mother's elder sister, stayed occasionally, often complaining of the cold but reinforcing my idea of the outside world as a splendidly exotic place. Her coming was heralded by the arrival, weeks in advance, of parcels containing great quantities of clothes. Often she would change her plans and the parcels would have to be sent on. She had travelled in the South Seas and would give me bright yellow cowrie shells from the lagoons, gaudy Hawaiian shirts on which were printed palm trees and lagoons, and records with Hawaiian guitar music. She was teaching me, without much success, to swim, saying that the first essential was for me to learn to float on my back. This was something I was reluctant to do because I had learned early on that, however picturesque the Irish coast, the water was bitterly cold. Extremely good-looking and with a strong mellow voice, Joan never married. She lived for many years in a cottage in Oban in Scotland with Monica Baldwin, a nun who had fled her convent after twenty-eight years and was a niece of Stanley Baldwin, the British prime minister before the war, with whom she exchanged frequent letters. Monica wrote a memoir, which did well, called *I Leap Over the Wall*, and was known in the family as 'The Show Jumper'. Aunt Joan had also written a book. It was about an expedition she had made up the rivers of British Guiana into the Amazonian forest looking for gold in 1930. Its title, *More Profit than Gold*, was a clear indication that she did not find any. I later saw photographs of her in pith helmet and semi-military brown uniform at her jungle camp with long canoes drawn up at the river bank. My mother, who had once made a language map in the forests of the Congo, spoke of Aunt Joan's expedition as a tragicomedy because it was the demise of her sister's most vigorous attempt to escape the predominant influence of her redoubtable mother.

Aunt Joan had pitched her camp on the edge of the forest canopy and was busily digging for gold, believing her mother to be safely distant in the Bahamas or Jamaica. Olive's father Sir Henry Blake had been governor of both islands and the family still kept up a connection. Then one day a canoe appeared around a bend in the river. It moved fast through the water and in the back, beating time for the oarsmen with her parasol, was my grand-mother, dressed like a Victorian lady in full regalia. She did not stay long. She said: 'Joan dear, I was getting a bit worried about you so I just thought I'd come to see how you were getting along. But I can see that everything is going splendidly.' She gave a few brisk instructions about re-pitching the tents to avoid drips from trees and, after a few hours, climbed back into her canoe to return to the mouth of the river. 'She never realised,' my mother would say sadly, 'that she had ruined poor Joan's bid for inde-pendence.'

My godmother Clodagh Anson also came to see us at Brook Lodge. She lived in a pretty but damp house, occasionally flooded by the river, on the Blackwater opposite Lismore Castle. It was owned by the Duke of Devonshire, to whom she was related. An intelligent and witty woman, she drove an elderly Volkswagen car at great speed. Every single birthday for forty years she sent me a cheque for one pound. She had, so I was told, almost killed me as a baby during my christening in St Mary's Collegiate Church in Youghal, holding me out with one hand like a butler presenting a plate on a silver salver. My mother rescued me before I fell to the floor.

Clodagh was brought up in a grand house near Lismore called Ballysaggartmore, of which only the elaborate gates now remain, but this had to be sold because of her father Claud's overenthusiastic investment in Russian bonds prior to the Revolution. His wife, Lady Anson, had gone to London and opened a soup kitchen and a shelter for down-and-outs close to her small flat near Putney Bridge. It was a curious upbringing for Clodagh. She remembered one resident, recently released from prison, always placing his little son's lunch on top of a wardrobe so the son could gain early experience in cat burgling.

Like Aunt Joan, Clodagh never married. She once told me that during the guerrilla war of 1919–21 her mother used to invite British officers from the garrison at Mallow to dinner in the hope of finding a suitor for her. The invitations were preceded by negotiations with the staff during which it was delicately underlined what a nasty blow it would be to the Anson family fortunes if any of the eligible officers were shot to pieces on the way from or to their barracks. Presumably they had the sense not to take the narrow dangerous road along the river from Mallow to Lismore too often because no marriage ensued. Clodagh did say that she had once received a proposal from a man, shy but otherwise suitable, which in other circumstances she might well have accepted. She was walking across a field with him in the penetrating Irish drizzle when one of her gumboots got stuck in the mud. She stood precariously on one leg, removed her other foot from the boot that was stuck and was tugging at it with both hands when he asked her to marry him. Rain trickling down the back of her neck, and trying not to topple into the mud, she abruptly turned him down and he never asked again.

Five

In the walled garden of Myrtle Grove are a pair of large cast-iron gates with two Chinese characters, each a foot high, attached to the thick bars. Round and black, the bars look like muscular snakes swallowing each other's tails. The gates appear wholly exotic amid the dahlias, roses and valerian, and they hang in a gateway cut in Youghal's ancient town wall. But they are not the only such gates in the world. An identical pair hang on the other side of the globe in a high brick wall, built to protect its people from bandits and pirates, surrounding the village of Kat Shing Wai on the Chinese mainland opposite the island of Hong Kong.

The surprising presence of the Chinese gates in Myrtle Grove was the result of the highly successful career of my great-grandfather Sir Henry Blake as a colonial governor at a moment when the British Empire was at the height of its power. Between 1898 and 1903 he was governor of Hong Kong, arriving just after the signing of a treaty by which the colony leased the New Territories on the Chinese mainland for ninety-nine years. These included the ancient village of Kat Shing Wai in the district of Kam

Tin whose people, all members of the powerful Tang clan, were angered by the British takeover and collected arms to fight the British occupiers as soon as they raised the Union Jack. Sir Henry, newly arrived in Hong Kong, ordered the army to crush the rebellion by the insurgent villagers.[1]

It was not a new experience for him. He had started his career as an officer in the Royal Irish Constabulary suppressing riots by Irish tenant farmers at war with Anglo-Irish and absentee English landlords. But by the time he reached Hong Kong, aside from his treatment of the people of Kam Tin, he had either mellowed or more likely he did not feel the same intense personal involvement as he did when defending the Protestant Ascendancy of which he was part. He liked the Chinese. His wife Lady Blake avoided the expatriate community by claiming to be ill when they called. Sir Henry refused to repatriate political exiles from Hong Kong to China, saying they would be tortured if they returned. An English-language newspaper in Ceylon, his next post, alert for any signs of weakening in imperial fibre, noted with alarm: 'In Hong Kong, Sir Henry Blake acquired a reputation, deserved or otherwise, of kowtowing to the Chinese. Some even went so far as to stigmatise him as pro-native.'[2]

Whatever Sir Henry's attitude to the Chinese as people, he had a demonstrable liking for Chinese furniture, ceramics and, as it turned out, gates. The uprising crushed – villagers said that 165 people were killed in the fighting – he seized the gates of Kat Shing Wai and shipped them back to Ireland where they were re-erected in the walled garden of Myrtle Grove, the house he had bought ten years earlier. A Chinese historian wrote: 'The end of the resistance and local villagers' failure was symbolised by Kat Shing Wai's iron gate which was taken by the British.' The episode does not seem to have made much impact on Sir Henry. He made a laconic note about taking over the New Territories in his diary on 'Monday, 17 April, 1899 . . . Place is handed over to the colony. Edith hoisted the flag . . . then the interpreter read my speech, which seemed to satisfy them . . . Afterwards distributed a pound worth of ten cent pieces to the children.'[3] There is no mention of resistance or how a party of military sappers had to blow a hole in the wall of the village to compel the Tangs to surrender. They were then forced to carry the gates and lay them at his feet as a sign of submission.

But the elders of Kat Shing Wai kept track of their gates and went to great lengths to retrieve them. Twenty years later they made representations to British officials, asking for their return. Sir Henry died in 1918 so they wrote to his widow making the same request. She either did not have the same predatory spirit as her husband or possibly she was uneasy over the peremptory means by which the gates had been acquired. In 1925 she had them taken down, crated up and sent back to Kat Shing Wai, where they still hang. A year later, shortly before she died, she received a testy phone call from Cork customs saying they had received a crate, so heavy that it had broken their crane, addressed to a 'Miss Blake, Ireland'. They asked her to collect it. When opened it was found to contain a perfect full-size copy of the Kat Shing Wai gates dispatched by the grateful elders of the Tang clan.

I visited Myrtle Grove frequently, usually taken there by Kitty, whose own house was close by in Church Street.

We went there because Shirley Arbuthnot, my first cousin, was one of the few children in the neighbourhood with whom I played. We could walk to Myrtle Grove because it was only a couple of miles from Brook Lodge. We first visited Kitty's house, which had an outer room of chilly formality with an enormous gold-coloured clock, and an inner room with a blazing fire where everybody sat cheerfully drinking cups of tea and eating cake. We would then walk up the street and turn right just before the entrance to St Mary's Collegiate Church into Myrtle Grove, which lay behind large wooden gates which were invariably closed. We did not go to the main house but across the front gravel to the nursery in a separate house where Shirley lived with her nanny Bessie O'Callaghan, Kitty's best friend. We played in the main room of the nursery which had a large bow window overlooking the street. Shirley, a pretty and strong-willed girl with brown hair, was in fact a year older than me, a slight edge in seniority which meant that she led and I usually followed. I was not very confident in dealing with other children because I had met so few of them. Shirley lured me at about the age of two to take part in a race across the floor still sitting on our potties. Seeking privacy for our competition, she locked the door of the nursery, forcing the gardener to rescue us by climbing through the window on a ladder. Soon afterwards our grandmother Olive Arbuthnot took us in her ageing car to a beach surrounded by rocky cliffs called Goat Island. Shirley ran fully clothed into the sea and I rushed after her. We were driven back to Myrtle Grove disgraced and wrapped in newspapers by an indignant Mrs Arbuthnot who refused to take us anywhere again.

I saw so much of Shirley in these years because of the friendship between Bessie and Kitty. Both were cheerful, intelligent, affectionate, came from Youghal and knew everybody in town. At other times Shirley was looked after by dour nannies from England and Scotland, often wearing uniform, who regarded the townspeople with fear and suspicion. Bessie had been preceded at Myrtle Grove by Nanny Burns, a grim figure who would present a carefully groomed Shirley once a day to her parents at 4.30 p.m. in the downstairs library of the main house. Bessie, who categorically refused to wear a uniform when she took the job, left Youghal to go and work in England some months before I caught polio in 1956, though it was anticipated that she would return. This unexpectedly turned into a much longer sojourn abroad in the USA after her Swedish employer in England, estimable in other respects, asked her if she would like a half or a whole potato for lunch. Potatoes were still central to the Irish diet and Bessie had been thinking of eating eight or nine of them. Realising that the cultural divide between the Swedish woman and herself was unbridgeable, Bessie took up the offer of a job in Chicago and did not return to Youghal for several decades.[4]

Myrtle Grove, behind its gates, was in any case somewhat cut off from the outside world. My uncle Bernard, Shirley's father, a former Royal Navy commander and captain of the Youghal lifeboat, was a good-looking, polite, gentle but reclusive man with a horror of casual visitors. This applied particularly to tourists, whom he called 'olishers', seeking to look at the house. Once he was lying on his back on the front gravel underneath a car trying to fix a defective part, with his legs protruding and with oil dripping on his face. At this delicate moment he heard a cultured English voice enquire: 'Excuse me, is this Sir Walter Ralegh's house?' Glancing sideways, he saw a well-shined pair of men's shoes and a woman's high heels standing beside the car. 'No,' he shouted back impatiently. 'It's *my* bloody house. Go away!' He immediately regretted his discourtesy and slid from under the vehicle to see Sir Harold Macmillan, the British prime minister, and his wife Lady Dorothy, scampering towards the gates.

Shirley and I spent most of our time in the gardens of Myrtle Grove. To one side of the front gravel there were the four enormous yew trees, so ancient that their branches had grown into each other. My mother told me that a visiting scientist had said the yews, which grew in a precise square and must therefore have been deliberately planted, were nine hundred years old. This would mean that they had been first placed in the earth before the Norman invasion, by the Danish traders and raiders who found Youghal an ideal port for their longships. There was a rough drawing of one of the ships cut into a stone in St Mary's Church. From a branch of one of the yews hung a swing on which Shirley and I would take turns sitting while the other pushed. I did not enjoy it very much because she would push me far higher than I wanted to go, so at the height of the swing Myrtle Grove would disappear from view and I, feeling slightly sick and clinging on tight, would peer into the upper branches of the yews.

Beyond the yew trees there was the main walled garden where the Chinese gates hung. Another entrance led into a pond garden with goldfish and rocks shaped like little rugged mountains, with miniature porcelain Chinese houses cemented into their slopes. Although Myrtle Grove was in the middle of Youghal it had five acres of grounds with stables at the back, its own museum, a croquet lawn, an apple orchard and a vegetable garden. There was even a long-abandoned brewery which the Blakes had half-demolished and turned into a Victorian Gothic romantic ruin. Alongside it they built a conservatory where a beautiful but poisonous white datura grew on the walls. By the time Shirley and I played there the romantic ruin was turning into a real ruin and chickens were living in the conservatory. When my mother was growing up in the 1920s thirteen servants had looked after the house and gardens, but thirty years later the number was down to two or three. My father caustically remarked that my mother's family had made a slight financial miscalculation sometime after the First World War in imagining that income tax was just a passing phase.

The main house at Myrtle Grove was very old, though far younger than the yew trees. It had been built in the late fifteenth century for the warden of the college of St Mary's Collegiate Church whose ancient stone tower, masked by trees, rose immediately behind the house. Protected by the town walls, it was not, like almost every other large Irish house built in Ireland at the time, designed primarily for defence. There were large windows cut through the massive walls. The builders, either because they were used to building military fortifications or because at the last moment they decided to take no chances on the Irish political climate, had made the walls ten feet thick where they faced the town walls and the hostile countryside beyond. Ralegh, mayor of Youghal in

1579–80, had enriched himself with land confiscated from the Irish at the end of the great Geraldine rebellion, in the course of which Youghal had been savagely sacked. Patrick Coppinger, the previous mayor of Youghal, accused of neglecting to keep the town walls in good repair, was hanged in front of the door of his own house. Myrtle Grove survived probably because the Earl of Desmond, who led the attack, used it as his headquarters. In the upstairs drawing room, about the richly carved wooden fireplace, was an Irish Sheilagh-na-gig, a delicate wooden carving of Celtic demigods, their legs splayed, celebrating rituals of fertility. It had presumably been taken from some church where Protestant reformers were ruthlessly culling such survivals, deemed pagan and obscene. On one side of the room was an oriel window where Ralegh's friend the poet Edmund Spenser, burned out of his own castle at Kilcolman, is supposed to have composed stanzas of *The Faerie Queen*.

Ralegh, drawn back to England by court politics, culminating in his long imprisonment and eventual execution, had not, in fact, spent a long time at Myrtle Grove. The house's unique personality – part Tudor, part Chinese – was the creation of Sir Henry Blake and his wife, Edith Osborne. Sir Henry's handsome, somewhat arrogant face, with piercing blue eyes and very dark hair, looked out from a portrait in the drawing room, almost a caricature of the successful colonial administrator. He had eloped with Edith, a great heiress, whose wealthy but ill-matched parents, having quarrelled bitterly for thirty years, came together briefly to disinherit their daughter. Lady Blake's portrait also hung in the drawing room, showing her dark, tough, Spanish-looking face. She was a keen and able artist, a botanist, a lepidopterist and a linguist, and bored by the tedious social round of a colonial governor's wife, she claimed to suffer from an incapacitating illness and painted hundreds of pictures of plants, animals and butterflies. I was delighted as a child by their exotic colours, but they also had the cool precision of scientific studies, made before botanists could rely on colour photography. These wonderful paintings covered the walls of the main staircase at Myrtle Grove as it rose two storeys and created the illusion that one was walking upstairs through a Caribbean paradise, alive with blue seas, exuberant green vegetation, leaping fish and dancing butterflies.

The Blakes had expectations but not much money when they bought Myrtle Grove from Sir John Pope-Hennessy, another colonial governor, for 1,500 pounds in 1894. Their plans to live there were in any case delayed because it came with two ladies in their eighties, the aunts of the previous owner, in residence. It had been agreed that they should continue to occupy the house until they died, something, it was tactfully suggested, that could not be long delayed. For several frustrating years the aged relatives did not take the hint, but when they finally did so the Blakes' fortunes had much improved. The house was soon filled with Chinese tables inlaid with mother-of-pearl, chairs with delicate scenes from the imperial court in Peking and vases with Chinese ladies standing gossiping by their tea houses. For a child it was like living inside an exotic doll's house which had come to life. There was a small white porcelain lady; when I stuck my fingers through two holes in the back they would stick out the front as if she had suddenly sprouted pink legs. I played with an intricately carved ivory ball, in which there were holes through which I could see other balls, also carved, each revolving freely inside, like worlds within miniature worlds.

When I was older I wondered if my mother had embroidered her accounts of the furious quarrels and embattled marriages of her family over the previous 150 years. But going by family papers and old newspaper clippings about the doings of the Osbornes, Blakes and to a lesser extent the Arbuthnots, it seems she had if anything toned down the details. No doubt the absolute but never unchallenged power of the planter aristocracy over the dispossessed peasantry made them prone to equally violent and extreme behaviour in their relations with each other. They had all arrived in successive invasions of Ireland. The Blakes had come by far the earliest on the coat-tails of Strongbow, the Earl of Pembroke, and the Norman invasion in 1169. They established themselves as merchants in Galway. The Osbornes and the Arbuthnots landed later in the sixteenth and seventeenth centuries when the Protestant Ascendancy, rich on the plunder of lands confiscated from the Catholic Irish, was establishing itself.

Powerful though they were in Ireland, the Anglo-Irish gentry were regarded in eighteenth- and nineteenth-century England as charming, feckless and untrustworthy. They were suspected of being on permanent lookout for rich marriages to supplement an uncertain income from their rack-rented Irish tenants. Thomas Love Peacock in his novel *Nightmare Abbey*, published in 1818, refers to a woman 'who had made a love match with an Irish officer. The lady's fortune had disappeared in the first year: love, by a natural consequence, had disappeared in the second:

92

the Irishman himself, by a still more natural consequence, had disappeared in the third.'

Three years earlier my great-great-great-grandfather, Sir Thomas Osborne, found himself the victim of English prejudice against Anglo-Irish gentlemen seeking marriage. A baronet with a large and beautiful house, Newtown Anner near Clonmel, he was a wealthy landowner with an income of about eight thousand pounds a year from his estates in Counties Tipperary and Waterford. He was also eccentric even by the tolerant standards of the Anglo-Irish gentry.[5] He had several thousand tenants on his estates, but he refused to accept rent in cash. Instead he demanded and received payment in kind. His tenants were forced to hand over chickens, sheep and cattle in payment for renting his land, something which had not happened in Ireland since the Middle Ages. He refused to dispense charity to the poor on his estates, but ignored it if they stole from him.[6] More sensibly he refused to be treated by any of the doctors in Clonmel and when ill always summoned the vet, on the grounds that he was more likely to know what he was doing.[7] But this strange man also had good taste. Although intensely antisocial – he would receive only three local families in his house – he rebuilt and greatly enlarged Newtown Anner between 1798 and 1802. It is unclear why he felt he needed a larger house since he was unmarried but, working with a local builder from Clonmel and without an architect, he created a stylish, spacious and comfortable house.

In the summer of 1815 Sir Thomas, now aged fifty-eight, visited Brighton, which was then highly fashionable. Not far from the sea the Prince Regent was building his oriental palace, the Brighton Pavilion, with its Mogul cupolas and Chinese interiors. Sir Thomas walked up and down beside the Steyne and visited the local circulating library. Here he saw and was attracted by a young woman, aged between nineteen and twenty and very good-looking, with dark raven hair and deep-set grey eyes. Her name was Catherine Rebecca Smith, and she was the daughter of a major in the Royal Marines from Rochester in Kent who had died three years earlier. Catherine had gone to Brighton together with two cousins called Sarah and Margaret Ward to stay with their uncle Mr Akers. At first the three young women, as they chose their books and talked, did not notice the intense interest of the ageing Sir Thomas. Catherine's younger sister Anna later wrote an astringent account of what happened. She says that Catherine was talking energetically to her cousins:

> She carried on the conversation, quite unconscious of the presence of an elderly gentleman who had been listening attentively to what had passed, and was so much pleased that he followed them out of the library and began conversing with them. After this he joined them every day, to the great annoyance of my cousins, who made it a rule to walk on each side of my sister as a guard, and greater still was their indignation when he walked into their box at the theatre uninvited.[8]

A week or two later a letter arrived from Sir Thomas for Catherine, proposing marriage. She was unenthusiastic and replied primly: 'I am sorry that my conduct has been so entirely misconstrued as to lead you to suppose

I had any intention of encouraging your addresses.' But as the months passed Catherine reconsidered, influenced, so her relatives believed, by the thought that Sir Thomas, a wealthy baronet, was a very considerable catch for a woman without any money of her own even if he was old enough to be her grandfather. Going by Catherine's letters she was intelligent, well-educated and unromantic, and at most felt a gentle affection for her ageing lover. Anna nurtured a certain resentment against Catherine perhaps because as a child she was dependent on her sister but also largely ignored by her. She wrote: 'My sister was a person entirely devoid of sentiment. Love, the one subject with girls when she was one, was a perfectly incomprehensible feeling.'[9]

Some of her family were horrified by her decision, though her mother approved the match. It was not only the great difference in age which worried them. The family solicitor in Rochester, drawing up the marriage settlement, found Sir Thomas's manner 'so very outré and singular' that he began to suspect that Sir Thomas was an Irish ne'er-do-well, lying about his vast acres, in pursuit of Miss Smith's modest competence. The solicitors interviewed him with unsatisfactory and worrying results. Questioned about the source of his supposed wealth, he could remember the names of neither all his estates nor his principal tenants. This was because both were too numerous to recall, but the solicitors for the Smith family were understandably convinced that the real explanation was their non-existence. When Sir Thomas could remember the names of his farms – Garrenmillan, Ballinagigla, Ballinasisla, Carigaready and Inchindrisla – they sounded bizarre to English ears. In letters surprisingly passionate for a law firm, the solicitors sought, ultimately in vain, to save Miss Smith from the embraces of the ageing baronet. Their enquiries did not go unnoticed. They had written to Lord Braybrooke, a friend of Sir Thomas, asking if Catherine's fiancé was indeed who he said he was, and Braybrooke replied that he was telling the truth about his fortune. Sir Thomas heard about the letter and was furious to discover that his credentials were considered suspect and had been investigated.

Even when reassured about his wealth, some members of Catherine's family fiercely opposed the marriage which was planned for April 1816. Catherine's brother-in-law wrote critically of the bride's mother that she was ready 'to run all risks and to let the sacrifice (for I cannot call it a union) be consummated on Monday next at Rochester'. He had no doubts that Catherine Rebecca herself had consented to the match for cynical reasons. He believed she was acting 'under a mistaken notion of female vanity and of future grandeur'. Sarah Ward, one of the two cousins with whom Catherine had met Sir Thomas the previous year, was still trying to dissuade her from marrying him up to the last moment. Anna says:

> All the Wards, especially Sarah, were indignant at the marriage, so much so that even while dressing my sister for the wedding, she said, 'Catherine, it is not too late, break off with Sir Thomas, and I'm sure Mr —— will be delighted to marry you.' Sarah was not clever.[10]

It did no good. The couple were married on 6 April 1816 in St Margaret's, Rochester.

Sir Thomas and Lady Osborne arrived at Newtown

Anner a month later on 8 May and at first she was enthusiastic. It was very different from Rochester. At least twenty-six servants had dinner every day in the servants' hall. In a letter home, she wrote that the house was 'immensely large; the hall very magnificent, supported in the centre by four pillars. Sir Thomas built the whole front of the house, and it does great credit to his taste. You could dance thirty couple in the drawing-room and dining-room, which are of exactly the same size.' But as the months passed Catherine came to see that her fantasy about the dance at Newtown Anner was never going to be realised. She complained to a friend in England: 'We are sometimes whole weeks without seeing the face of an acquaintance; and such is the haughty reserve which Sir Thomas keeps up in the neighbourhood that, with a few exceptions (only three I believe), I can call on the families once a year, no more, even should they persevere in visiting me.'[11] She read omnivorously, swam in the Anner river and kept a pet bullfinch. Half a century later Catherine's daughter Catherine Isabella said that Sir Thomas, 'though he loved her with a fervour', was used to intense solitude and did not realise that this sort of existence 'depressed and withered' his young wife.[12]

There were other problems. Catherine was astonished to learn of Sir Thomas's immensely cumbersome system of getting paid in kind for letting land. She wrote in amazement that he insisted 'on being paid in young horses, cows and pigs'.[13] The tenants did not like it and sometimes land could not be let at all. Catherine also objected to what she saw as the Irish habit of winking at petty theft and preferring it to more regular charity for those in need. Catherine Isabella said acidly that there was a saying around Newtown Anner that '"Sir Thomas was a rail gentleman." If he saw a man drive off his colts along the road (meaning stealing them), he would look the other way.'

Overall, Catherine was lonely but not unhappy. Anna, her sister, then aged eight or nine, was sent to Newtown Anner for two years to keep her company but she recalled many years later that Catherine ignored her. Anna was left to wander through the gardens 'overgrown with weeds as high as I then was myself'. At first she would talk to the gardeners, but when Sir Thomas saw her doing so he said it was never to happen again. She was deeply bored, and her only comfort was reading books from half a century before which she found mouldering in a box. Anna says Sir Thomas 'was kind to me, playing at games and even dancing, till one evening, unfortunately, I announced I did not like dancing with an old man, it frightened me, so that was given up'.[14]

Catherine became pregnant soon after her marriage and had a son called William, whom she adored, and two years later Catherine Isabella was born. Sir Thomas died in 1821. His wife found that people had started to plunder his property even while he was on his deathbed. She fought off in the courts an attempt by her co-executors to put the estate in chancery. But she was devastated when William died suddenly at the age of eight (Anna says he died because of excessive bleeding by the local doctor, thereby showing the wisdom of Sir Thomas's reliance on the vet). She turned to religion, and many of her letters are to Protestant clergymen. Part of the hall was curtained off as a chapel. Her sister wrote: 'There never was a week but what some meeting was held in the hall at Newtown, or prayers in the evening with very long addresses.' After breakfast Catherine would sit by an open window and give money to beggars who came to talk to her. She even attempted to convert the Roman Catholics of Clonmel to Protestantism, creating deep resentment. Once, after a Protestant meeting in the town, Catherine was hit on the head by a stone hurled by an angry Catholic but was uninjured because it hit a large knot of her hair and only broke the comb holding it in place. A local priest stopped her carriage being thrown into the river.[15] But she was not entirely illiberal. She wrote in a letter in the late 1820s on the eve of Catholic Emancipation: 'You know how strong my Protestant feelings are – so strong that I am constantly tempted to treat popery with opprobrium and contempt; but I do not agree with you wishing that emancipation should be withheld.' Brought up in England, she was uncomfortable with the bitter religious divisions of Ireland. She found it a great trial 'that my own footman refuses to join in my family worship as an unholy thing. That the man who eats my bread, looks upon me, who really feel an anxiety to save my own soul and the souls of others, as a heretic, sinking into perdition.'[16]

She ran the estates efficiently, sketched continually and began to learn ancient Greek. She was highly intelligent and well-educated. She wrote letters in Italian and French as well as English. She records at one moment: 'I have given up "Homer" as not good for the mind; and instead of translating a heathen poet, I have found profit in every way in learning the Gospel of St Luke by heart in Greek.' By the 1830s her income had increased even further because of revenues from copper mines at Bunmahon in County Waterford. She started three schools and during the Famine employed starving farmers to landscape the grounds of the house as a means of providing work (though there is something chilling about famished peasant farmers trying to stay alive by digging artificial lakes, romantic vistas and even a wooden Doric temple).

She devoted much of her time to bringing up Catherine Isabella, the heiress to Newtown Anner and the Osborne properties since her brother William's death in 1824. Catherine Isabella was brought up in great luxury. When she came of age on 3 July 1839, a dinner was held for 1,400 tenants followed by dancing, fire-balloons, fireworks and bonfires blazing in celebration on the slopes of the nearby Comeragh mountains. One of those attending, a certain Captain Chaloner, wrote a poem commemorating the party of which one verse reads:

> The long, long dance in endless files
> Was cheered by high-born Beauty's smiles
> For midst the rustic maze
> The graceful Heiress oft was seen
> Gliding along the velvet green
> To Erin's ancient lays.[17]

The use of the word 'Heiress', capitalised in the original text, is significant. From the age of six, when her brother died, Catherine Isabella knew she was extremely rich. Treated as a princess by her adoring mother, she not surprisingly grew up egocentric and emotional. She would switch from deep affection to intense hatred with disconcerting speed. She was easily moved to jealousy and had an abiding and not unreasonable suspicion that people were after her money. Her attitude to men, particularly to potential husbands, mystified her aunt Anna Phipps who in 1880 wrote notes about her niece's love life as she had observed it. She gave them to Edith Osborne, Catherine Isabella's elder daughter, who had by this time quarrelled bitterly with her parents. Anna explained to Edith: 'Your mother's manners to gentlemen were so very cold, it was difficult to judge in any particular case what her feelings were.'[18]

Catherine Isabella was pursued by a number of suitors and not only for her money, since some were just as rich as she. In the early 1840s Anna recorded that Catherine Isabella and her widowed mother had gone on a visit to Italy 'with three servants and a carriage and two ponies'. In Naples she became engaged to a Prince Trecasi. 'I believe he was the only man she ever liked.' Unfortunately the prince was in line of succession to the throne and the appalling Ferdinand II of the Two Sicilies, universally known as King Bomba after bombarding his own rebellious people, and reputed throughout Europe for his brutality, insisted that the marriage should not take place unless the children were brought up as Roman Catholics. Since mother and daughter were active Protestants, this was impossible. The engagement was broken off and they returned to Paris. Both women must have seemed good catches. They were introduced 'to one of those men who frequent clubs and pass their time in card playing and smoking; he was not young. I suppose he thought in marrying L.O. [Lady Osborne] he would have money for some years, but her daughter was most indignant when she found out what was going on. She told me, that going in to the room where they were arranging their plans, she attacked the man most violently and insisted on all being given up, which it was.' Back in London Catherine Isabella received a proposal from a Sir Jacob Preston, who had a house in Ireland. She announced the engagement to her mother immediately, saying: 'I have accepted Sir J.P. and I wish I was dead.' She and her fiancé quarrelled and their plan to marry was abandoned.

Soon afterwards, in 1844, Catherine Isabella met an English MP and former soldier called Ralph Bernal, who proposed and was accepted. He agreed to change his name to Bernal Osborne to maintain the family name. In later years his wife and eldest daughter came to detest him so much that his true character is a little elusive. Osborne got poor reviews in my family because of the role he played in disinheriting my great-grandmother. He came from a family of Spanish Jewish merchants who had moved to Amsterdam to escape persecution and then to London in the eighteenth century where they converted. Their money came from plantations in the West Indies. Ralph Bernal's father, also called Ralph, was a Whig MP from 1818 to 1852 and reckoned he had spent 66,000 pounds on fighting elections. He was also a collector and when he died in 1854 his vast collection, crammed into his house in Eaton Square and one of the most famous of its day, was auctioned off for 71,000 pounds. The sale of portraits, furniture, porcelain, faience, enamels, metalwork, ivory, glass and armour took thirty-two days. When his father remarried in 1832, after his first wife had died, Ralph was forced, much against his will, to join the army where he spent much of his time writing comic verse – a habit which never left him. Contemporaries found him witty, good at electioneering and lightweight. They said his failure to get a job in the government, though he was an MP for constituencies in England and Ireland from 1841 to 1874, was due to laziness 'and the absence of that sobriety of judgement which is dear to the average Englishman'.[19] Disraeli, a friend of his, described him, rather patronisingly, as 'the chartered libertine of debate'.

There was much more to Bernal than this. He complained, in words that my father would have sympathised with, that his funny stories had led him to being taken less seriously than he deserved. 'I wish I had never uttered a joke in my life,' he said. 'If only you came to learn what my jokes have cost me.' As an English MP he opposed the way in which Catholic tenants in Ireland were forced to subsidise the Protestant Church of Ireland. He was attacked by Protestant no-Popery gangs. He fought ferocious election campaigns. A poster from an election in 1852 in Middlesex warns voters: 'Beware of Osborne the Advocate of Papal Aggression.'[20] He complained: 'I have been constant but the constituents have not been constant! It has been my fate to be turned out of a great English constituency for my Irish predelictions; to have crossed the water to an Irish constituency and to have been turned out of an Irish constituency for my care of the English connexion.'[21]

Right up to the last moment there was a chance that Catherine Isabella would change her mind about marrying him. Anna Phipps gave Edith, the elder of the two daughters produced by the marriage, a vivid account of the day of the wedding which was to lead to such misery for all concerned. She wrote:

On the morning of the wedding I went early, and going into your mother's room, I found her sitting before the glass, her hair being dressed, while she

103

was involved in finishing a piece of worsted work she was determined should be done before she married. I went with her in the carriage. I do not know why. When the ceremony was over and while some little difficulty arose from Mr Bernal not having brought any money, which however Col Phipps fortunately had, your mother and I sat down in the vestry and having nothing better to do we both burst into a violent fit of crying.

The day did not improve. At the wedding breakfast an obscure cousin gave an embarrassing speech and Anna wondered why Benjamin Disraeli, another guest at the wedding, soon to become leader of the Tory Party and famously eloquent, had not been asked to speak instead. The happy couple then went off for the first night of their honeymoon in the castle of a friend. This too did not go well. 'I do not think that the female character was well understood by Ralph Bernal for the next morning Mrs O. told me he left her to call on some friends, leaving her alone all day.' They travelled to Ireland. Almost immediately Ralph Bernal's behaviour began to grate on his new wife. Tenants from Newtown Anner had gathered to greet them but their coach was late because Ralph Bernal Osborne, as he now was, out of meanness or lack of money, would use only two horses. His adoption of his wife's name seems to have provoked an identity crisis. On occasion he would revert to his old name. One of his first acts at Newtown Anner was to have all the sheep rebranded with the initials R.B. (Ralph Bernal) replacing C.I.O. (Catherine Isabella Osborne). Anna concluded: 'I think, small as these things were, they mortified your mother.'

Six

Catherine Isabella and Ralph Bernal Osborne, came to detest each other. They had two daughters, Edith, my great-grandmother, born in 1846, and Grace, born in 1848. He was by now MP for Middlesex and stayed mostly in London while his wife lived largely in Ireland bringing up the two girls. When he did visit Newtown Anner Catherine Isabella often greeted him by saying: 'I trust you are well, Mr Osborne, and how did you leave your mistresses?'[1]

It was not an easy childhood for the two daughters. In 1880, just after her mother died and when relations with her father were particularly bad, Edith wrote what was, for a Victorian lady, a peculiarly frank and chilling account of her home life:

From almost my earliest recollection I remember my father and mother being on bad terms. When I was very young indeed I recall one day at my grandmother's bedroom at Newtown. My mother was very angry and excited and was complaining to my grandmother about my father and my grandmother asked her if it would not be better if they were to separate. I do not think I understood at the time what she meant. The most violent scenes used frequently to take place between my parents, my sister and I often stood holding each other's hands in the corner very much frightened and not knowing what it all meant. My father generally wished we should be sent out of the room, but my mother would desire us to remain as she wished us to see how she was treated. My father was a great deal away from home and my sister and I always remained with my mother who was usually very kind to us and indulged us much more than my father did. She often told me how happy her life had been before she married, how my father had wrecked and ruined her life and how he would ruin our lives too if he could, but that she would never leave it in his power to do so and would save us from him. I hated my father and looked upon my mother as a suffering angel who would protect us from him.[2]

Photographs of Edith in her late teens show her as having a tough, resolute face, looking somewhat older than her years. There is also a hint of restlessness. In 1872 she published a well-written book, beautifully illustrated with drawings by herself, called *Twelve Months in Southern Europe* about her travels through Germany, the Austro-Habsburg Empire and the Mediterranean. She was accompanied only by a lady's maid and a young cousin who was a clergyman. It is not the work of an inhibited Victorian girl. At one moment she complains vigorously about a hotel in Constantinople which had told her that there was a public baths next door. In fact it was some distance off, compelling her, she notes with irritation, to walk through the streets in her dressing gown.[3]

Catherine Isabella, despite the episode of the rebranded sheep, kept control of her own wealth. She had a persistent need to feel that she could give orders to those around her, notably her own daughters. Edith recalled: 'One day she called me and said, "Remember, Edith, if I die tomorrow you can turn your father out of the place if you like, everything will be absolutely yours."' On other occasions she would threaten to disinherit her daughters if they displeased her, saying she had the legal right to leave everything to her footman if she wanted and they would have only five thousand pounds each. Edith found her mother did not like to be contradicted: 'If in any argument or discussion any one agreed with me and did not take her view she sometimes was very angry and said they were worshipping the "rising sun" but that I was absolutely in her power.'

Catherine Isabella carried her hatred of her husband to extraordinary lengths. When Edith was sixteen or seventeen her mother wrote a novel called *False Positions* which was published anonymously in 1863. It was a thinly disguised attack on Bernal Osborne, who was one of the chief characters in the book, and her family tried to persuade her to suppress it. Edith said the novel created even more hostility between her parents: 'I did not read the book till long afterwards but I was greatly annoyed about it as I understood that it would expose a great deal of dirty linen to the public.' This presumably refers to Bernal Osborne's affairs. A break-up between the warring couple was often talked about and a deed of separation was drawn up even before Edith was born, but never acted upon. Edith says she herself proposed 'a regular separation which I thought would be in the interests of everyone'. But Catherine Isabella, when angry with her daughter, would 'tell my father that I was doing all I could to separate them and this of course vexed him very much as he never spoke to me about affairs as my mother did'.

Going by Edith's account, it seems her parents, though intelligent, cultured and well-educated, were invariably a nasty and demented couple when it came to relations with each other. They quarrelled about everything from the purchase of a property – Catherine Isabella wanted it in her name and Ralph wanted it in his – to his decision, to which she strongly objected, to stand as MP for Waterford. Sometimes the reason for a particular quarrel was obscure to the children. During one violent scene, which Edith witnessed when she was very young, 'My mother was very much excited and threatened to tell "the children" some circumstance which it was evident my father did not wish us to hear for he stopped her, saying if "she dared" he would tell us something else.'

It is curious to look at bucolic photographs of this deeply unhappy family. Surprisingly, there are many wonderful pictures of the Osbornes and Newtown Anner in the 1850s taken by W. D. Hemphill, a surgeon in Clonmel who was a close friend of the family. He was an extremely able photographer who also grew orchids, collected Waterford glass and was a skilled ivory-turner. The Osborne women evidently liked being photographed and even posed for him in fancy dress. In two pictures Edith, who must have been in her late teens, is dressed first as a peasant from Styria and then as a peasant from Rome, roles not out of keeping with her dark appearance. A picture of startling beauty taken from the dining room of Newtown Anner looking towards the mountains in about 1860 shows Catherine Isabella in a full Victorian gown looking down at Edith or Grace sitting on the grass wearing a white hat with a ribbon. Behind them is a mowing machine drawn by a horse and tended by two men, and two women gardeners with brooms for sweeping up leaves. In the middle distance are tall deciduous trees and beyond them the hazy outline of the Comeragh mountains. The drawing room of the house, also photographed by W. D. Hemphill, is less attractive because the Bernal Osbornes redecorated it in fussy over-ornamented Victorian style after the death of Lady Osborne in 1856.

Because of the furious rows over the three marriages contracted by Catherine Rebecca, Catherine Isabella and Edith in the course of the nineteenth century, I find it easy to forget that they were all accomplished women. Catherine Rebecca made Newtown Anner something of an intellectual centre visited by the Swiss landscape artist Alexandre Calame and the English watercolourist and engraver Thomas Shotter Boys. As well as her anonymous attack on her husband, Catherine Isabella brought out a two-volume collection of her mother's letters. From their private letters, the three women come across an extremely well-read; they also wrote precisely and elegantly.

Given Catherine Isabella's obsession with controlling the lives of those around her and her fear of fortune hunters, there was also bound to be trouble when her daughters came of marriageable age. Edith recalled that her mother had once remarked to her, '"I can always prevent you marrying if I like by my money power." I said "You know that would never influence me." She answered "I don't believe it would influence you but I don't believe a man exists whom it would not influence." I replied "If such a man does not exist then I certainly shall never marry."'

Antipathies in the Osborne family exploded spectacularly in 1869. Grace, elegant and pretty compared to Edith's dark looks and determined square face, wanted to get engaged to a Mr Ross whom she had met when the family was visiting Oxford. At first all had seemed to go well. They met again in London. Family visits were exchanged. After speaking to Mr Ross at a cricket match at Lords, Catherine Isabella exclaimed: 'There's a young man I can understand a girl being in love with.' The Osbornes and the Rosses went to Hamburg to take the waters. Edith, knowing her own family, did not think this was a good idea. Suddenly Catherine Isabella became hostile. Bernal Osborne, despite their sulphurous relations, had not lost all influence over his wife. Edith said: 'My father was not civil to them and I have always thought he set my mother against them.' Mr Ross proposed but Grace was too frightened to tell her mother. She asked Edith to do so. Catherine Isabella objected strongly. 'The upshot was that my parents would give my sister nothing and they did not consider he had enough money,' Edith recorded. 'Accordingly there was to be no marriage.'

The following evening Grace allowed Mr Ross to escort her back to the house where the Osbornes were staying. Edith returned a few minutes later:

When I opened the drawing-room door I came upon a fearful scene. I thought my mother had gone perfectly mad. She was holding my sister pounding her against the wall in a perfect frenzy and using the most terrible language calling my sister every kind of name. My sister was very white and exhausted. She said to me 'She is mad.' I at once took my sister from my mother, stood in front of her and told my mother she must not touch her. My father then burst into the room in an equally mad state of frenzy. He cursed and swore at me.

It turned out that Catherine Isabella had met Grace and Mr Ross at the door of the house and had struck him before dragging her daughter upstairs. Nor did the affair end there. Bernal Osborne challenged Mr Ross to a duel, though he was later induced to withdraw it. The marriage, needless to say, never took place.

This frantic scene in Hamburg was the last straw for Edith. 'I was so dreadfully annoyed at the whole affair that I said I could not continue to live under my parents' roof after the manner in which they had treated me and the language they had used to me.' She refused to speak to her father. She told friends in Paris of her resolve to leave home. Her mother, acting sensibly for once, suggested a compromise whereby Edith would live in a house they owned called Carrigbarahane House in County Waterford some miles from Clonmel, and visit her parents at Newtown Anner. Edith says: 'I finally agreed to continue to reside with them on condition of their acknowledging me to be a perfectly free agent and not interfering with me in any way.'4

*

111

Edith, knowing her parents, cannot seriously have expected them to stay out of her life. The furious row over Grace's engagement to Mr Ross was repeated, though with a different conclusion, when Edith met a good-looking and recently widowed police officer called Henry Blake who commanded the Royal Irish Constabulary (RIC) in the nearby market town of Clonmel. Once again it was Catherine Isabella who initially made the running. She sang duets with the young inspector and invited him to stay at Newtown Anner. 'I think I never saw my mother so charmed with any one as she was with Mr Blake,' Edith later wrote. 'She raved about him to many people.' She was surprised when her mother suddenly took against him and blamed malicious gossip. In fact, Catherine Isabella's alarming switch in emotional gear from deep liking to sustained hatred was typical of the way she had behaved to people throughout her life.

There are differing accounts of exactly what happened next. My mother believed that Edith simply eloped with Henry Blake, climbing down a ladder from her bedroom window at Newtown Anner. She then took refuge with another Anglo-Irish family called Bagwell, who lived not very far away at Marlfield House on the other side of Clonmel, and was married three weeks later. The Bagwells and the Osbornes never spoke again. Possibly the elopement was more complicated and drawn out. First the Osbornes tried to persuade Edith not to marry the young police officer, whom they denounced as an adventurer and a former draper's assistant from Limerick. By one account she agreed to wait for two years, during which she would travel abroad, but after that, if she had not changed her mind, she would marry Henry Blake whether

her parents liked it or not. Observing the row, Anglo-Irish neighbours had a coarser explanation for Catherine Isabella's rage. They believed she found Blake highly attractive compared to her philandering husband. Clodagh Anson, my godmother, said: 'You know my mother used to say that the particular shock and anger of Mrs Osborne at the elopement was not only due to Blake's inferior social and financial position, but to the fact that he used to visit Newtown Anner where she herself and he used to play duets on the piano together and you know what *that* means.'[5]

Henry and Edith married in 1874 and she was promptly disinherited. Bernal Osborne, though barely on speaking terms with his wife, came rushing back to Ireland to support her in casting off their daughter. In true Victorian fashion they forbade her name ever to be mentioned in their house again and even added a clause to their wills saying that no descendant of Mrs Blake should inherit any of their property. At the same time their sense of social disgrace must have been mitigated since their second daughter Grace had married earlier in the same year William de Vere Beauclerk, the tenth Duke of St Albans. The Duke was a descendant of Nell Gwyn, Charles II's favourite mistress of whom he famously said: 'Don't let poor Nelly starve.' He was well off – he owned seven thousand acres in Nottinghamshire and Lincolnshire – rather than spectacularly wealthy and was a crony of Bernal Osborne, who left him all his papers in his will. When Bernal Osborne died at Bestwood, the St Albans house in England, in 1882, the Duke wrote a laudatory preface for a privately printed biography of his late father-in-law.

The newly married Blakes were poor compared to Edith's previous palatial standard of living. Henry resigned from the police and became a Resident Magistrate first in King's County (now Offaly) in central Ireland and later in Tuam in Galway. These were dangerous jobs. The land war had reached a new phase of intensity. With the foundation of the Land League in 1879 it came close to a general uprising. Charles Stewart Parnell was reinvigorating the Irish Parliamentary Party. Resident Magistrates like Henry Blake were hated as the men who oversaw evictions, arrests and trials. An open grave was dug in the lawn of their new house in Tuam. My mother always said that Edith Blake was at heart an Irish nationalist and a friend of Parnell's sister Anna. There is probably an element of wishful thinking in this. An article in a sternly Unionist newspaper called the *World* highly commends Blake for his ruthless repression of rioters and gives a vivid picture of the home life of the Blakes in Tuam in 1881. Its correspondent reported favourably on his entertainment, commenting that at times 'the guest quite forgets the revolver lying on the side-table and the heavy shutters closed and barred against the possibility of a potshot from without'. He added that Mrs Blake acted as her husband's bodyguard, accompanying him everywhere. Once she had saved his life when she overheard in court a whispered plot to kill him on his way home. 'She is always armed, a dead shot with a pistol and practises every day,' says the reporter admiringly.[6]

Edith found other uses for her gun. The bitterness between the Blakes and her parents remained deep. Just how angry Edith felt about being disinherited became clear after her mother died on 21 June 1880 at the age of sixty-two. The Blakes made a pre-emptive strike, possibly intended to contest her will, by taking over Carrigbarahane House, Edith's bolthole ten years earlier. Then on 25 June they went to Catherine Isabella's funeral, a grand affair attended by most of the gentry of the area.

When they returned to Carrigbarahane, however, they found that the agent for the Osborne estate, Captain Tottenham, had used their absence at the funeral to break into the house by smashing a window and thereby regain possession. Captain Tottenham then departed, leaving the house in charge of a caretaker named Edmund Thrump.

The Blakes found Thrump in the kitchen. Henry seized him by the collar and began to wrestle with him to force him out the door. Edith drew her pistol and shouted: 'Look at this – if you don't go out I will put what's here through you.' Later in court Henry produced the rather lame defence that Edith was not intending to shoot Thrump because he, Henry, was standing between her and her intended victim and she could not have got a clean shot without endangering her own husband. Frightened, Thrump fled the house. At this point the Blakes seem to have realised that they had gone too far. Edith sent a message to his home apologising and enclosing half a sovereign. Henry still seems to have believed that he could cling on to the house, saying there were no legally appointed trustees for the Osborne estate. Seeking to conciliate Thrump, he said: 'Before two days you will be caretaker of mine and Mrs Blake.' In other words, Thrump would not be out of a job and should keep this in mind when giving evidence about what had happened.

Henry had put himself in a very dangerous position.

The following day he was accused before Stradbally petty sessions court of using 'force and violence' to expel Edmund Thrump. Edith was charged with threatening to shoot him with a revolver. In defending himself Henry, evidently still furious, made the charge, reported verbatim in the papers of the day, that the whole affair had been cooked up by the Duke of St Albans, whose wife Grace was now about to inherit the Osborne estates. He said: 'The only one who has an interest in this matter is my noble brother-in-law the Duke of St Albans, and if he has anything to do with it, I tell him that it is an ignoble and discreditable thing for him to bring Mrs Blake here.' He told the magistrates that if he was fined so much as a penny by them the Duke would go to the Lord Lieutenant to demand his dismissal from his job as a Resident Magistrate.

There is an air of desperation about Henry's defence. He claimed that Edmund Thrump had condoned what had happened by accepting half a sovereign. He explained that the initial takeover of Carrigbarahane House by himself and Edith was justified because there were no trustees for the Osborne estate: 'It therefore devolved upon the eldest daughter of the late Mrs Osborne to look after the property.' It was not a convincing case. His strongest card was probably that he knew the magistrates who decided whether to send the case to trial. One of those described by the local paper as sitting on the bench later wrote in to say that he had been there, though not in his official capacity but as a friend of the accused. Probably the magistrates did not want to get involved in a notorious family feud. They dismissed the case.[7]

*

Sir Henry was lucky that the crisis over the Osborne inheritance happened when it did. By the autumn of 1880 agitation against landlords and in favour of Home Rule was testing British control of Ireland to a degree which had not happened since the rebellion of 1798. Parnell and most of the Irish Parliamentary Party would soon be in jail. It was not a good moment for government to lose one of its more efficient and ruthless officials. In 1882 he was further promoted, in the renewed crisis after Lord Frederick Cavendish, the incoming Lord Lieutenant of Ireland, and his under-secretary T. H. Burke were knifed to death by an Irish militant group as they walked across Phoenix Park in Dublin. Blake was appointed one of five Special Magistrates in charge of restoring order by almost any means possible under the Coercion Act which followed the killings. He was given command of all soldiers and police in six of the most disturbed counties in west and central Ireland.

He was well-qualified for the job in terms of character, family, religious and political background. The Osbornes were wrong to think that he came from an entirely humble background, though his family was poor. The Blakes, numerous in Galway since the Norman invasion and partly Gaelicised in the Middle Ages, were petty landowners living in fortified tower houses across the county. In the turmoil of the late sixteenth and seventeenth centuries some, sniffing the political wind, turned Protestant while others remained Roman Catholic. Henry Blake acknowledged as an ancestor Sir Richard Blake who had been speaker of the Catholic Confederate Parliament in Kilkenny at the height of the savage wars in the 1640s. But his own branch of the family, the Blakes of Corbally,

117

became Protestant, giving total loyalty to the Ascendancy, which they were to defend to the end. Unlike the more aristocratic Osbornes and Arbuthnots, their estates were small or non-existent and they had few family or financial connections with England.[8]

When the Irish Constabulary – it only acquired the title Royal some years later – was founded earlier in the century, Peter Blake, Henry's father, sold his land and joined the force. He acquired a fearsome reputation and was notorious for commanding his men to fire into a crowd in the early 1830s, killing seventeen people (though by one account he was lying wounded on the ground at the time and may not have personally given the order to shoot). He ended up as overall inspector for the RIC in County Limerick. Henry, born in 1840, became a police cadet in 1859 and served in almost every county in Ireland. A pro-government newspaper in Dublin records him suppressing a riot in Tipperary town at about the same time that he was visiting Newtown Anner to sing duets with Mrs Osborne and, more covertly, to woo her daughter. The paper reports that a tall figure suddenly emerged through a shower of stones and shouted: 'Stop throwing stones this instant or I will fire! Throw one more stone, and I give the word to fire and clear the street.' The correspondent, who going by the tone of his piece, seems to have regarded all Irish peasants as cowardly and sub-human, only deterred by the guns of the police, claims to have heard a voice in the crowd exclaim in alarm: 'It's Blake of Corbally; and the father of him shot down the people and so will the son.'[9]

Henry Blake was more than a brutal gendarme of an occupying power. He wrote lucidly and well in defence of the Ascendancy of which he was part, usually employing the pseudonym – he was, after all, a government official – Terence McGrath. In 1880 he explained in an English magazine, St James's Gazette, that 'there are two Irelands, more clearly defined in religion, feeling and interests than were the Northern and Southern States of America in 1864'. He saw no bridge between the two nations, one Protestant and the other Catholic. He asserted: 'It can never be too often repeated that Ireland must be governed either by Irish ideas or English ideas.'[10]

The Anglo-Irish gentry in their decline after Irish independence are sometimes portrayed as befuddled victims of history, perhaps getting a rather better press than they deserve. This is in part because so many of them – a remarkable number for such a small community – wrote eloquently and affectionately in novels and memoirs about the doings of their ancestors. Unfortunately Henry Blake was much more the typical Anglo-Irishman of the nineteenth century than William Butler Yeats. At the height of their power the Anglo-Irish gentry and their hangers-on were as brutal, violent and racist as any colonial elite defending its interests anywhere in the world. Henry Blake, for instance, opposing a government measure to alleviate the condition of Irish tenant farmers in 1880, wrote: 'It is not a demand for fair rents, but a declaration that landlordism in any shape is robbery; and rather than rent be paid the virtue of the bullet must be tried.'[11]

The phrase about the bullet was more than just a figure of speech. The New York Times wrote that, after two years as an all-powerful Special Magistrate, Blake 'made himself so fiercely hated by the people that he had to be removed from Ireland'.[12] The government clearly felt it owed him. Even so his pay-off in 1884 was particularly munificent. He was made Governor of the Bahamas and given a knighthood. This seemed to some at the time to be excessively generous even for services, however dangerous, rendered by Sir Henry in maintaining British rule in Ireland. My mother suspected that his rapid promotion as an imperial administrator was the doing of Grace, Edith's sister, and now Duchess of St Albans. The bitter animosity over the Osborne inheritance and the scuffle in Carrigbarahane House four years before, when Henry believed the Duke was plotting to have him sacked from his job, had died away. Bernal Osborne, whom Henry and Edith loathed, had died in 1882. A few years later Sir Henry is recorded as showing the Duke around newly purchased Myrtle Grove. My mother believed that 'Grace had always loved her sister and felt guilty that she had everything while, in a worldly sense, Edith had nothing'.[13] Edith was not exactly penniless but, as shown during the row over Mr Ross in Hamburg, she was the tougher of the two daughters and had always defended Grace from her mother and father.

The *New York Times* correspondent in London had no doubt about the reasons behind Sir Henry's rapid promotion. After three years in the Bahamas he was briefly made Governor of Newfoundland, which he and Edith found too cold. He was then offered the Governorship of Queensland in Australia. This provoked a furious reaction from numerous Irish immigrants in the colony. Leaders of both political parties in Queensland sent cables expressing astonishment and indignation over the appointment. The

(*Below*) Sitting in a howdah on Jacky, led by my mother.

(*Right*) Me in 1955.

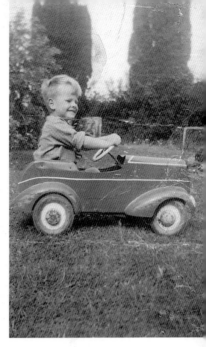

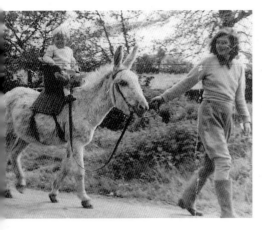

(*Left*) Andrew and I on the way to school in a trap pulled by Blackie the horse.

(*Below*) Me in 1956, just before I got ill.

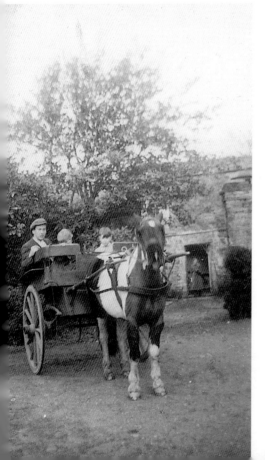

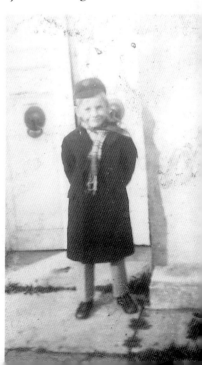

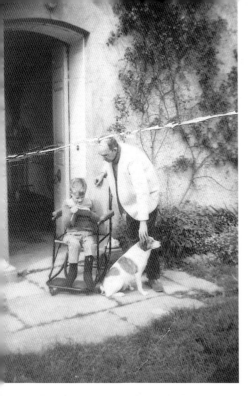

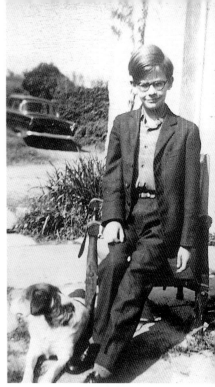

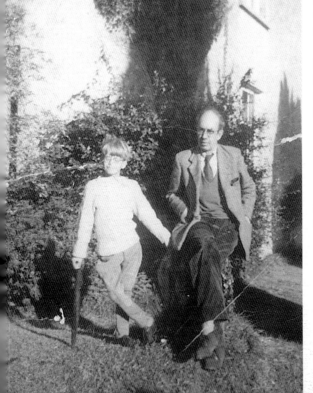

(*Above left*) Aged seven, with Claud and Charlie the dog, outside Brook Lodge.

(*Above right*) Aged eight. Unable to stand, I have to hold on to a chair for a photograph.

(*Left*) With my father at Brook Lodge.

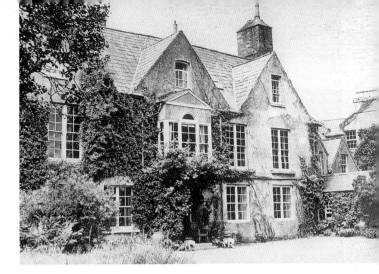

(*Above*) Myrtle Grove, once the home of Sir Walter Raleigh.

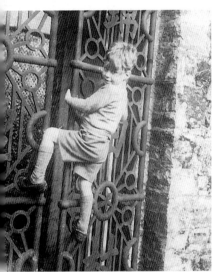

(*Left*) Climbing the Chinese gates looted by my great-grandfather Sir Henry Blake.

(*Below*) Kitty Lee, my nanny, at the front gate of Brook Lodge.

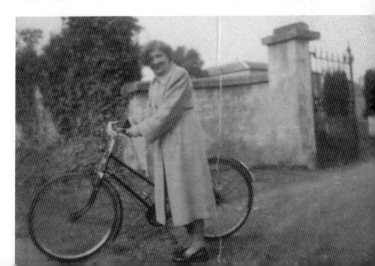

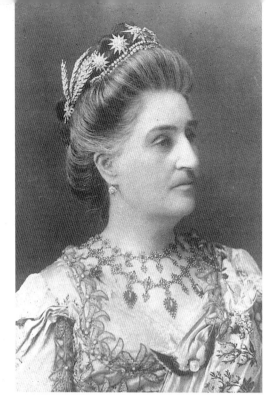

(*Left*) Edith Blake,
my great-grandmother.

(*Below*) Edith Blake (far left)
and Henry Blake (far right)
at their daughter Olive's wedding in Hong Kong in 1903.

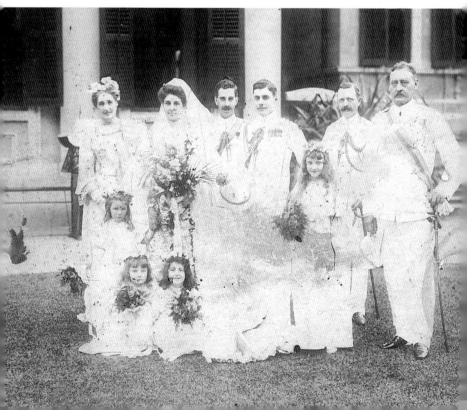

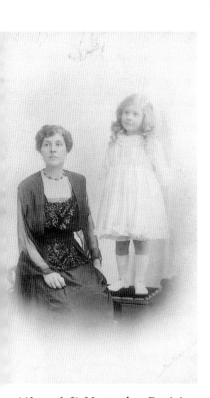
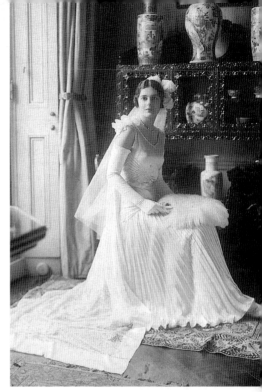

(*Above left*) My mother Patricia as a girl, with her mother, Olive Arbuthnot. (*Above right*) My mother as a debutante, 1931. (*Below*) In the 1970s.

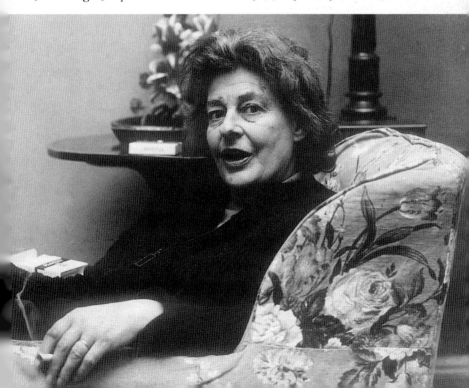

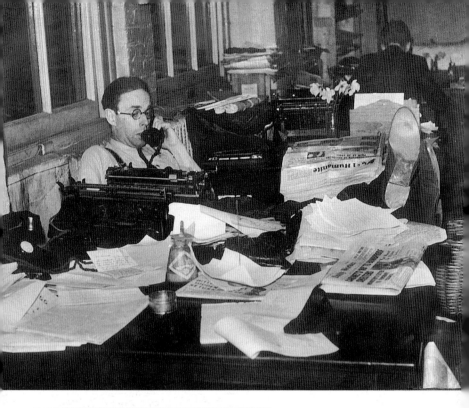

(*Above*) Claud Cockburn at the office of *The Week*.

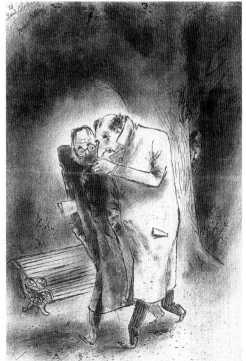

(*Left*) James Fitton's cartoon of Claud Cockburn and John Strachey.

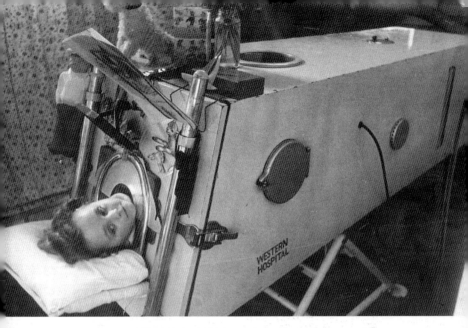

(*Above*) A child in an iron lung.

(*Below*) St Finbarr's hospital today.

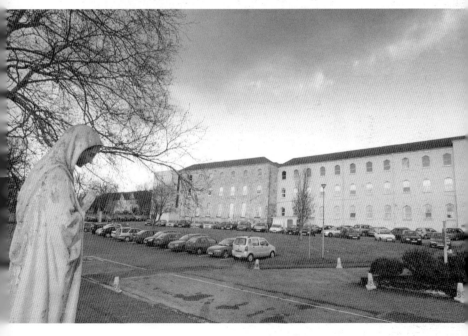

(*Overleaf*) Claud Cockburn (centre) at *Private Eye* with (back row)
Christopher Logue, Peter Cook, Christopher Booker; (seated) John Wells,
Richard Ingrams; (front) Gerald Scarfe, Tony Rushton.

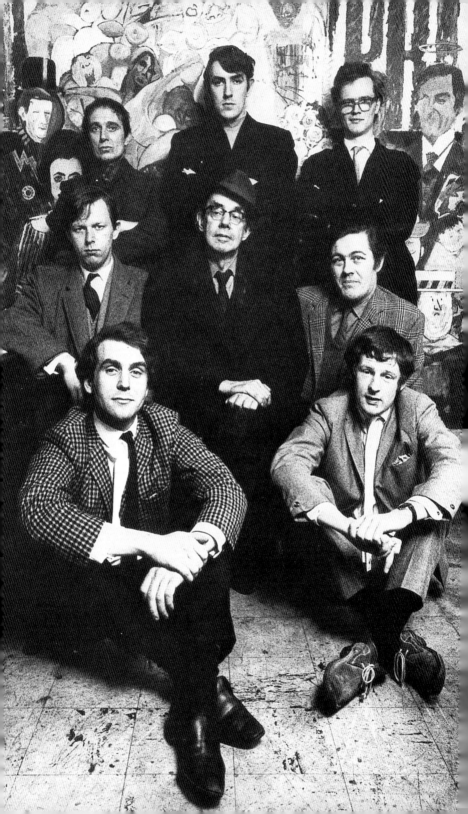

newspaper, possibly briefed by Irish nationalist MPs, was singularly well-informed about the background to the affair. Its correspondent wrote:

> Blake, who is one of the numerous landlord family of that name in Connaught, was seven years ago a poor sub-inspector in the Irish constabulary, but a handsome young fellow, who ran away with and married the elder daughter of Bernal Osborne. Her younger sister had just before wedded the Duke of St Albans, and by the influence of this ducal connection Blake was made one of the five district magistrates on whom the coercion act of 1882 devolved.

This later point probably is not true because Blake was already highly regarded by the government as a Resident Magistrate. But his rapid rise in the imperial civil service was no doubt helped by his connection with the Duke, a Liberal under Gladstone who defected to the Tories after the Liberal leader proposed the Home Rule Bill of 1886. It was the time of the great split in the Liberal Party, precipitated by the crisis over Ireland. The newspaper goes on, with surprising vehemence, to explain that 'when the Duke of St Albans ratted from Gladstone as a Liberal Unionist a part of the price he secured from the Tories was Blake's advancement to the Governorship of Newfoundland and now the effort is being further made to promote him to Queensland'. It expected, however, that such was the wave of criticism that the government would have to withdraw an appointment 'that is resented by every Irishman in Australasia'.

It was a delicate moment for the Tory government. It

had just taken the dangerous course of trying to end Parnell's career by accusing him of secretly writing letters supporting violence and terrorism. It was an attempt which was about to explode spectacularly in their face when the letters were exposed as crude forgeries. Further controversy over Sir Henry's appointment was not welcome. A few weeks later in the House of Lords, Lord Derby, who had appointed Sir Henry Governor of the Bahamas, said 'he was one of the ablest men he ever met'. But at the same time it was announced that the governor designate had asked to be relieved of the appointment.[14]

Sir Henry did not do badly out of the affair. He was appointed Governor of Jamaica instead. At the request of the inhabitants he was asked to stay for a second term so ended up serving there from 1889 to 1897. Edith produced some of her best pictures there, minutely observed watercolours of Caribbean plants and butterflies at all stages of their existence. For instance, one day in 1892 she painted a female giant sphinx moth she had reared. It is an elegant picture of the moth at various stages: as a caterpillar feeding on the leaves of a plant, as a chrysalis and finally as a fully formed moth taking wing. Some two hundred of her watercolours from Jamaica, a small part of her output, were later presented to the Natural History Museum in London where they are conserved.

Away from the toxic political climate of Ireland, Sir Henry showed himself a benign and humane administrator. In Jamaica he campaigned against labourers being recruited to build the Panama Canal, distributing posters warning that, however attractive the wages, they stood a good chance of dying of malaria. Indeed, he seems to have taken on board at an early stage the discovery that it was the bite of the mosquito that infected victims with malaria. As Governor of Ceylon, his last post which he was given after leaving Hong Kong, he searched out ancient documents to try to show that it was the Sinhalese who first realised the connection between the mosquito and malaria. He thought that this would make anti-mosquito measures more acceptable. When he retired in 1907 a local paper in Colombo noted perceptively that Sir Henry's 'natural gifts would have appeared to have fitted him more particularly for ruling over diverse races rather than people composed exclusively of his own nationality'.[15]

Neither of the Blakes was a racist. In Hong Kong they preferred the company of the Chinese to the local expatriates. They were particularly close to a fabulously wealthy Chinese businessman called Sir Robert Ho Tung, the son of a Dutch sea captain and a woman from Shanghai. At the age of eighteen he had become the Chinese business agent of Jardine Matheson, the Scottish trading firm which had helped found Hong Kong. He then went into business on his own account. The factor which first brought Sir Henry and Ho Tung together was probably opium. The government in Hong Kong depended on the 'opium farm' for a large part of its income, renting it out to the highest bidder. Several months after he had arrived in Hong Kong, there is an interesting note in Sir Henry's diary dated 29 March 1899. It records: 'Ho Tung is prepared to give $300,000 a year for a five-year term of opium farming . . . 2½ chests [about 450 pounds] a day consumed here.' Social relations were close. Ho Tung later visited the Blakes in Ireland. It was all in sharp contrast to the behaviour of another British governor of Hong Kong who vetoed an attempt by Sir Robert to rent a house on the Peak, the Nob Hill of Hong Kong reserved for whites only, saying that it would be impossible to have a 'half-caste with four wives' living there. When Ho Tung funded a school, he was subsequently told that there was no question of Chinese children being allowed to study there.[16]

After his stint as Governor of Ceylon Sir Henry returned to Ireland in 1907 to live in Myrtle Grove. He remained a man of great energy, reconstructing the grounds of the house. He vigorously opposed Home Rule and was attacked by the local newspaper, the *Cork Examiner*, which correctly said his opposition was based on 'the intelligent anticipation that the passing of the Home Rule Bill will synchronise with the passing of Ascendancy rule in Ireland'.[17] He died in 1918, a few short months before British rule began to crumble. Edith lived on another eight years. She had long given up painting because of deteriorating eyesight and she devoted much of her time to bringing up her granddaughter, my mother Patricia – the rest of her family had decamped to England – and ignoring the War of Independence and the Civil War by now raging across Ireland.

Edith showed her determined character up to the end. The vicar of St Mary's Collegiate Church angered her by sawing off a branch which had grown over his churchyard but came from a tree in the garden of Myrtle Grove next door. Edith was infuriated that he had cut off the branch without asking her permission. She decided to boycott his graveyard and persuaded a bishop to consecrate part of the Myrtle Grove orchard. It was here that Sir Henry was buried in 1918 and Edith was buried beside him eight years later.

Seven

Inscribed above the door of a substantial grey stone building opposite Kitty's house in Church Street were the words 'Protestant Asylum'. I was embarrassed by this. I knew about asylums because Kitty had pointed out to me the mental asylum, known as 'The Mental', on top of a steep green hill by a quarry overlooking the road into Youghal. I had not then come across the word used in the sense of refuge and I was embarrassed because I knew there were few Protestants in our town. Their scanty numbers were all too visible when we attended St Mary's Collegiate Church at Christmas and Easter and looked at the rows of empty pews. I was worried about so many of our tiny community suffering from mental illness that they required an enormous building of their own. I could not read the words above the door but they were in large capital letters and Kitty read them out to me. I wished that, if there were so many Protestant lunatics in Youghal, we had not gone to such lengths to advertise the fact.

The gates of St Mary's were at the top of Church Street. The church was vast. It stood, grey against the green hill behind, just outside the walls of Myrtle Grove. Several cannon on the town walls on top of the hill pointed out over the town. Inside the church gates a path ran uphill past to the enormous east window of the church. In a plot of green grass just below it, beside a monkey puzzle tree, were the graves of my grandparents, Jack Arbuthnot who died in 1950, the year I was born, and his wife Olive, who died three years later. St Mary's was the size of a cathedral rather than a parish church, ludicrously big as there were only a couple of hundred Church of Ireland Protestants in Youghal as compared to five thousand Roman Catholics. On Sunday I could see crowds after Mass surging out of the Roman Catholic church a few hundred yards away. There had to be half a dozen Masses in the course of the day so everybody could find a seat. St Mary's had been built seven hundred years earlier, after the Norman invasion, when Youghal was a prosperous port serving the newly arrived settlers from England and Wales. In the Middle Ages there had presumably been enough worshippers to fill the church, but since the Reformation it had been a symbol of Protestant power and wealth. The tombs and plaques of local Anglo-Irish gentry, often recording their achievements and sometimes their demise in obscure colonial wars, lined the walls. In the south transept towered the magnificent tomb of Richard Boyle, Earl of Cork, a highly successful Elizabethan adventurer, with painted sculptures of himself, his two wives and some of his fifteen children. I was given bad reports of him as a child, being told, falsely by all accounts, that Boyle had betrayed Sir Walter Ralegh by buying his Irish estates for a pittance in return for a promise – which he failed at the last moment to fulfil – to help him avoid prison and execution.

128

Small the Church of Ireland congregation may have been, but it maintained its social divisions. The Arbuthnots, as patrons of the living, had the right to sit in a gallery, reached by a narrow wooden staircase, at the far west end of the church. We were often late, a fact made obvious to other worshippers by the loud creaking of the stairs as we climbed them, the sound reverberating down the almost empty nave. I was deeply bored by the services, and spent much of my time looking for bats. My mother had told me that as a child she had rescued baby bats which fell into the gallery from the rafters high above. It seemed an exciting way to pass the time. Several times I brought a matchbox and looked hopefully upwards, but the bats must have moved elsewhere and I had to abandon my rescue mission.

I did not listen to, and if I had would not have understood, the sermons. They were in any case difficult to hear given that long distance between us and the rector standing in the pulpit at the far end of the nave. This was a pity because for several Christmases in the early 1950s, so the family told me later, these sermons were fraught with interest. The congregation was made up of a score or more of local gentry and their families, but most of the people, the backs of whose heads we could see in the first few rows beyond a sea of empty pews, were substantial shopkeepers. Many of the bigger shops and workshops – though none of these were of great size – were owned by Protestants. At one time this might have benefited shops seeking to supply the British garrison, which had a barracks in Youghal up to 1922, or the local gentry. But thirty years later the shopkeepers' adherence to the Protestant faith did them no good at all. As a dwindling

129

minority they might have expected a few words of encouragement and good cheer at Christmas from their rector, the Reverend Watts. Instead, so my brother Alexander recalls, they had to endure wounding criticism from his lips:

> Peering down from his pulpit at the shopkeepers who were making a couple of shillings out of the Christmas buying spree, Watts would savagely denounce the gross commercialisation of a holy festival celebrating the birth of the Saviour. Then he took to attacking the atom bomb and the shopkeepers saw their chance. They complained to the bishop and Watts was demoted and became curate of Watergrasshill, a desolate hamlet twenty miles inland.[1]

Some of the congregation may have been surprised to see my family in church at all. They may have surmised that my father was an atheist and my mother, though sympathetic to many Christian tenets, was not a believing Christian in the traditional sense. My father regarded going to St Mary's as largely a cultural activity of the Anglo-Irish which he was happy to go along with for a couple of days a year to please my mother. 'I may be an atheist but I am a Protestant atheist,' he would declare jovially. 'I don't see why disbelief should be a barrier to religious bigotry.' My mother took it all more seriously, seeing St Mary's and the Church of Ireland as part of her Anglo-Irish heritage of which she was extremely proud. In later years, living in the village of Ardmore five miles from Youghal, she repeatedly frustrated attempts by a bishop to close down the little Protestant church for lack of attendance by ensuring, any time he attended a service, that it was packed with her Roman Catholic friends. Religious enthusiasm in any case was never part of the Anglo-Irish tradition. My uncle Bernard, a foe of enthusiasm of any description, played a role in choosing new rectors for St Mary's and would seek to weed out candidates displaying too much fervour. 'I thought he was a bit religious,' he declared of one potential incumbent. Many years later he apologised to me for offering me a dubious-looking glass of sherry, saying: 'I call it "bishop's sherry" and it's pretty nasty. I got it specially to give to bishops so they don't come too often.'

Anglo-Irish weddings were much like those in England but christenings and funerals were longer affairs, usually with plenty to drink. My mother's christening in St Mary's had been peculiarly prolonged for another reason when the Bishop of Cork recoiled at giving her the names chosen by my grandmother. The names Olive had given to her other five children were traditional enough but when she came to my mother she decided on something more exotic. When the bishop asked how the baby should be named her godparents responded in unison: 'Kawara, Finnbaragh, Evangeline.' It was never clear where Mrs Arbuthnot had got the first name. One theory held that it was a waterfall in New Zealand which she had seen and admired, and another that it was the name of Lord Kitchener's sister who was a friend of hers. The bishop insisted that the first two names would have to go. Ignoring my grandmother's pleadings, he pointed out that my mother had been born on 17 March, St Patrick's Day, and called her Patricia.

By the time I was growing up there was no animosity between Protestants and Catholics in Youghal, but there was a deep sense of difference. As was usual in Ireland, religion, class and national identity were mutually reinforcing. After all, many people in Youghal had English names and were presumably descended from so-called 'Old English' settlers in the Middle Ages who had remained Roman Catholic and were persecuted as such after the Reformation along with the native Irish. There was another reason for the lack of friction between the two religions in Youghal. Sir Henry Blake had said, while the outcome was still in doubt, that Ireland was going to be 'governed by Irish ideas or English ideas' and added that for him the former meant Roman Catholic ideas. By the time I was growing up it was obvious who had come out the winner in the struggles of the previous hundred years.

But even in my short life the barriers between the two religions had become less rigid. Andrew and I both went to the Loreto convent in Youghal without anybody showing surprise. The only difference between us and other pupils was that we were not allowed to attend scripture lessons because the nuns worried they might be accused of trying to convert us. When Andrew and I caught polio they closed the school for three days so staff and pupils could pray for us. Only a few years before, Alexander's education had provoked significant controversy. He was aged six when my parents came to Youghal in 1947. They saw no reason why he should not be sent to the Loreto. But my grandmother immediately rebelled at the idea. She was not a bigot but to her traditional mind, the gulf between the two religions was unbridgeable. She pointed out that there was a small Church of Ireland school in Youghal at the far end of town. It was, unfortunately, about to close because its numbers had dropped below seven, the minimum required by the Church. My grandmother set to work, like an Irish-American politician getting out the vote, to recruit more children for the school. Protestant shopkeepers who supplied Myrtle Grove were firmly told that their children must attend the moribund little school. Some pleaded the difficulty of getting their children there. My grandmother purchased a donkey and trap which was kept at Brook Lodge. It would first pick up Alexander and then do a round of the town collecting other little Protestants and delivering them to the school.

The atmosphere in Youghal was deeply Roman Catholic, as it was in the rest of Ireland, with an intensity of religious belief seen probably nowhere else in the world. It gave people an ability to endure and in Youghal in the early 1950s, impoverished and with a sense that Irish independence had made no difference to their plight, there was a lot to be endured. A hundred yards from Alexander's Church of Ireland primary school, opposite the Devonshire Arms hotel, there was a shrine which was a symbol of the strength of religion in our town, though perhaps not in the way originally intended. It was built to celebrate the declaration of the Dogma of the Assumption, the belief that the Virgin Mary did not die but was assumed into heaven, by Pope Pius XII in 1950. Beneath a statue of the Virgin the builders had run out of space for the inscription. The result was that the first line read 'Dogma of the Ass', and the second continued 'umption of the Virgin Mary'. My parents wondered, with some merriment, what archaeologists of the future would conclude about religious practices in Youghal in the mid-twentieth century if the second line of the inscription was destroyed and only the first survived. In other less devout countries the inscription might have been replaced with one less likely to attract derisive comments from the profane. But in Youghal there were few if any profane enough to joke about the statue or its strange inscription, which remained unchanged for more than half a century.

Once, when a winter storm combined with a particularly low tide in Youghal Bay, I was taken far out on to the sands to see the dark red trunks of trees, half buried by the sand. They were part of a drowned forest of yew trees, submerged by the incoming sea in some prehistoric catastrophe. We brought some of the ancient yew branches home to Brook Lodge and they slowly dried to a dull pink. They did not survive long. My father felt permanently cold and one day, forgetting how old the wood was, he threw it on the fire where it burned with a light blue flame. Even after the sea inundated Youghal Bay yew trees must have survived on the hills around the mouth of the Blackwater river. The name Youghal – *Eochaill* in Irish – means yew wood. But by the time I was growing up the only yews surviving in town were in the grounds of Myrtle Grove where Shirley and I used to play.

Youghal owed its existence as a small port to the Blackwater and the Atlantic, but it had a precarious relationship with both. The river was difficult to navigate at low tide when the retreating water exposed banks of soft grey mud. The old stone quays offered little protection against south-east gales. A few years later my uncle Bernard's two-masted schooner, the *Three Brothers*, was torn from its anchor by a storm and wrecked on the front strand. Part of the town was built on land reclaimed from the estuary and during spring tides the water sometimes penetrated the alleys around the town centre. Wooden boards and putty were kept ready to protect doorways. But it turned out that the sea had not stopped its work of erosion after engulfing the ancient yew forest so many centuries before. One day a woman walking with her dog up the road beside the sea leading from the Loreto convent to the lighthouse suddenly disappeared. The pavement on which she was standing had collapsed, and she and her dog fell twenty feet. It turned out that for years the sea had been sucking out the foundations of the road, also the main highway along the south coast of Ireland. As lorries and cars thundered over the solid-looking tarmac, a large cavern was being formed a few feet beneath their wheels. Investigators later said they could see the bottoms of telegraph poles protruding through the roof of the cave. The woman was knocked unconscious by her fall but her dog squeezed through a narrow entrance to the cave on to the beach below and attracted attention by barking. The road was closed, forcing drivers to skirt the town centre, and for days afterwards concrete mixers poured cement into the cavern.

People in Youghal were embarrassed by the collapse of the road and the temporary disappearance of the woman and her dog. They sensed it was the sort of slightly ludicrous disaster that English people liked to hear was happening in Ireland. People in town were ambivalent about the antiquity of the buildings around them. A little of this stemmed from the fact that its most famous monuments – Myrtle Grove and St Mary's Church – were symbols of foreign conquest. Even the elegant clock tower, built in the late eighteenth century, through whose arch ran the main road to Cork, had once been used as a jail and served as a convenient spot for the execution of rebels. A hundred yards away was the old water gate known as 'Cromwell's Arch', through which, after ravaging the country, Oliver Cromwell had departed for England in 1650. At the other end of town were the Tudor almshouses, built for the poor of Youghal by the Earl of Cork. He was particularly keen that they be used to house former soldiers who had helped him in his career of conquest.

Youghal was picturesque because it was poor. The Industrial Revolution reached this part of Ireland late in the day. It had been in a state of slow decline since the Famine. Little new had been built in town over the previous half-century. Paddy Linehan, the tall, gaunt owner of the Moby Dick pub, a butcher's shop and later chairman of the local council, recalls: 'In 1946 I and some other young fellows agreed that we had our freedom all right, but we didn't have freedom from want, from hunger, from unemployment, from malnutrition. There was tremendous emigration.'[2] Many men took jobs in England, repairing bombed-out buildings. Others had earlier joined the Irish army during the war. 'You could tell they were malnourished because before they went off the backs of their necks looked hollow but after six weeks their necks would fill out and look round.' By the time I started going to the Loreto convent this was beginning to change. Opposite the greyhound track and not far from the sea front a businessman from Cork called Bill Dwyer had opened two textile factories called Seafield Fabrics and Blackwater Cottons. When Andrew and I were driven to school in a gig or a trap, the streets were full of horses and carts, providing enough business for two blacksmiths. But within a few years cars replaced horses. Wages were low enough to attract industrialists. In 1954 John Murray started a small carpet-making factory called Youghal Carpets in an eighteenth-century warehouse. In its first year it employed just four workers but soon 850 people in Youghal were earning high wages there and others were being bussed to the factory from other towns along the coast and up the Blackwater. The prosperity did not last very long. Just as workers in Ireland would work for less than those in England, so twenty years later there were countries from China to Brazil where the pay was even lower than in Youghal. Entry into the European Community in 1973 left the local factories open to competition. Paddy Linehan also blamed the luxuriant lifestyle of the factory workers at Seafield Fabrics and elsewhere. 'They had *coloured* lavatory paper,' he told my brother Alexander. 'It was like the Shah of Iran.'

Others in Youghal, aside from Paddy Linehan, wondered what could be done to rescue the town from its slow slide into decay. When Kitty Lee and I walked into town from Brook Lodge the road took us past a large stone farmhouse in which lived Tom Casey, editor of the *Youghal Tribune*, a local paper with a circulation of around a thousand. Alexander used to go ferreting with his son. The *Tribune* mostly stuck to lengthy reports of funerals and sporting events but every few months Tom would write a leader entitled 'Wake Up Youghal!', invariably giving grave offence in the small town. Once, after his wife had asked him to choose a less controversial topic for his next piece, he had almost been shot. He had written a laudatory piece about Youghal's one notable guerrilla action in the War of Independence. It had been a typical attack with a roadside bomb, as lethal to British soldiers in Ireland in 1921 as it was to US troops in Iraq in 2004. The monthly report of the County Inspector's Office in Cork on 2 June 1921 has a succinct summary of what happened:

> On 31st ult. at about 8.25 a.m. 100 men of the Hampshire Regt, with their Colonel in charge, marched with their band from the military barracks at Youghal to their rifle range via fixed route. When they got to a place called Summerfield Glen a landmine exploded killing three outright and wounding 22 other, 3 of these died shortly afterwards. The mine was connected to an electric battery by about 150 yards of cable. It is believed that there were only two men involved in carrying out this outrage. They were seen running away from the scene. They were fired on by the military but escaped.[3]

Also typical of such incidents, whether they take place in Youghal or Baghdad, is that the soldiers under attack open fire in all directions. In this case they shot at a horse-drawn vehicle, wounding a Roman Catholic priest called Father Roche, and killing the driver and horse.[4]

Shortly before Tom Casey's article appeared two men stopped him on the road near his house. One of them levelled a pistol at his chest. They said they had heard about his forthcoming article and wanted it withdrawn. Their reason was peculiar but compelling. The men who had really blown up the soldiers had since died. The two threatening Tom, although originally from Youghal, had had nothing to do with the original ambush. So far from fighting for Irish freedom they had in fact been serving with the British Army in India at the time. But they had fraudulently applied for state pensions, claiming to be the members of the old IRA who had carried out the attack (members of the old IRA who had fought in the war of independence before the establishment of the state were eligible for pensions). They pointed out to Tom that if his article appeared with the real names of the ambush party they would lose for ever their chance of receiving their pensions. Rather than face an impoverished old age, they were prepared to shoot him.

The inhabitants of Youghal, a town hoping to encourage tourism from Britain, were ambivalent about advertising too overtly the sufferings of Ireland under British rule. One particular problem was the statue in the Green Park outside the Adelphi Hotel overlooking the mouth of the Blackwater. In the years immediately after the war the first tourists to return were from Britain and most of them had recently been in the British armed forces. But if they crossed the road from the Adelphi they were immediately confronted by a statue of Father Peter O'Neill, a local priest, and on the plinth inscriptions in large letters recalling that he and three other men had been either 'cruelly flogged' or 'unjustly hanged by British soldiers in 1798'. The visiting British tourists objected strongly to this, claiming the British Army would have done no such thing. Paddy Linehan consulted my father on how the inscriptions might be changed to avoid offence and he suggested writing the same words in Irish. In the event the inscriptions have stayed in English to this day.

On our side of town there were a number of new council houses opposite a row of ancient cabins. I was interested in the new houses because I had been told a story about an elderly man who lived in one of them and had got into trouble because he tried to help his next-door neighbour. She was even older than he was and nearly blind. He would read her the local paper, the *Cork Examiner*, every morning. But he became bored by its relentlessly upbeat account of local affairs and began to invent stories of greater interest. All went well until he pretended to read out a story that a man in Cork city had been arrested for strangling an elephant in his cellar. When the old lady complained to her neighbours about the cruelty of people in the city, they responded with disbelief and derision and his small invention was unmasked. As I walked past the house I imagined the man struggling with an elephant somewhere in a cellar beneath my feet.

The centre of Youghal stretched for a couple of hundred yards on either side of the clock tower. We went to Merrick's, the main drapers, which I liked because the shop assistants would put the money paid by customers, together with the bill, inside a hollow wooden ball. This would then run along a system of overhead rails to the main cashier. The cashier would unscrew the ball and send it on its return journey with the change and a receipt inside. Sometimes we had a specific mission in mind such as getting my hair cut. This took place at the barber's owned by a man called Mr Fox who advertised himself in his shop window as 'the man with the educated fingers'.

On visits to Youghal with Kitty Lee we went either to the streets around her house or to the beach. The latter was usually the 'near strand' below the road which, unbeknownst to us, was being silently hollowed out by the sea. When I went with my parents, visits to town had a different objective. My mother would go to the shops and my father to one of the larger pubs which had a working phone and which he could use as an office. Around the middle of the 1950s he mostly used the Wright House on the far side of the clock tower. It was from here that he telephoned St Finbarr's to find out if Andrew and I were alive or dead. There were about thirty other pubs in town and at one time or another my father must have visited them all. He was a popular visitor, not least because his radical past attracted those who felt his presence injected a certain amount of drama into the situation. One of the smaller pubs he visited was Cooney's, just before Church Street, a very small pub even by Youghal standards. Moss Cooney, the son of the owner, remembers being allowed as a treat when a child to peek through the door from the kitchen at 'the dangerous man' – my father – who was standing at the bar.

Occasionally we would go to Horgan's cinema, one of the few places of entertainment in town aside from the pubs and a dancehall called Red Barn, which I had vaguely heard of as a place of debauchery. Films in Ireland were heavily censored at the time. Anything which looked like a kiss or an embrace was immediately excised. Anything to do with violence was left in. Sometimes Maisie Horgan, the friendly woman who ran the cinema, would find that the soundtrack was interfering with her conversation with her friends. She would abruptly turn the sound down so the six hundred people packed into the cinema would have to strain to hear the rest of the whispered dialogue. When I was four there had been a grand screening at Horgan's of *Beat the Devil*, the film directed by John Huston based on my father's novel. I must have been considered too young to go, or at least I do not remember the film. Alexander reported that the people of Youghal, not entirely without reason, found it incomprehensible but applauded heartily, none more so than the bailiffs and other representatives of the commercial sector of the town.

Eight

Aside from Myrtle Grove, the nearest Anglo-Irish mansion to Brook Lodge, close enough for us to drive there by horse and trap, was Ballynatray. It was a large yellow eighteenth-century house four miles away from us on a bend in the River Blackwater, with dark green woods behind it and a soggy green field with coarse grass and bulrushes in front. My mother was a childhood friend of Horace Holroyd-Smyth, the son of the then owner Rowland, whose family had owned the estate since late Elizabethan times. The approach to the house was a little hazardous. We had to take a right turn off the main road through one of the lodges, now abandoned and with bricked-up windows. We then got out of the trap and led the horse forward because the drive to the house passed over a wooden bridge made out of old railway sleepers with gaping holes in it through which we could see the muddy water swirling below. We drove another mile down the drive through the trees, past a second ruined lodge engulfed by enormous rhododendron bushes so dense that they shut out the light, until we reached a hill covered in bracken and alive with leaping deer. Just beyond was the house with paint flaking off it and two giant pillars behind which were the main doors. Once inside I was impressed by great antlers of the extinct Irish elk – twelve feet from tip to tip – dug from some bog and hung high up on the wall of the front hall. They were only dimly visible in the murk because there was no electricity at Ballynatray. Horace and his parents had abandoned parts of the house, too cold and too dark to live in, and used one or other of the smaller rooms as a sitting room. At this age – I must have been about four or five years old – I did not really distinguish between the personalities of the people I met and the houses where they lived. Horace was a gentle, friendly, rather retiring man, but I thought of him as being part, and not the most important part, of Ballynatray. I cannot remember now what he looked like. But I can still recall the giant elk antlers as well as a portrait of Sir Walter Ralegh, with a slightly sinister look on his face, in court dress hanging in the front hall.

In a clump of trees opposite Ballynatray were the grey ruins of a monastery called Molana Abbey, built on an island in the middle of the river in the sixth century and now connected to the land by two long dykes. They were not very effective at keeping the river back. Close to the driveway there was a grove of dead white trees killed by the salt in the water which rushed in one night when the bank of one of the dykes collapsed. We went on frequent picnics to Molana, spreading blankets on the grass beneath a nineteenth-century statue of the saint who founded the monastery. Sometimes we ate beneath the east wall of the nave which leaned precariously over a path leading to a fish weir, built by monks a thousand years before, where

144

we caught whitebait and flat fish. As the tide went down the fish were funnelled by nets attached to wooden posts into a shallow pool. We would wade through the grey, oozing mud with shrimping nets and buckets to the weir, surrounded by herons and seagulls crowding around the pool filled with thrashing fish.

At first sight Ballynatray, romantic and decayed, might have appeared to be a symbol of the Anglo-Irish gentry in the years of their decline: the half-abandoned mansion, the lack of electricity and the gardens turning into jungles. Around it were other monuments to successive waves of conquest overlooking the dark water of the river. Looking south from Molana Abbey we could see Temple Michael, a medieval stone keep covered in ivy and inhabited only by crows, founded in the distant past by the Knights Templar. Beside it was a Protestant church, its interior walls painted light blue, overlooking a cemetery with a locked mausoleum covered in green moss where Holroyd-Smyth ancestors lay buried. Horace was trying to keep the church open by holding services, presided over by a clergyman who arrived on a motorcycle once a month, and attended only by Horace, my mother and myself.

But Ballynatray was not really typical of the Anglo-Irish in the 1950s. Few, if any, of the other large houses on the banks of the Blackwater were without electricity at the time I was visiting them for picnics and tea parties. Nor had the fate of their inhabitants been particularly harsh. A guidebook to the Blackwater, written just before the Famine in the 1840s, shows that most of the Anglo-Irish families living there then were still there a century later. There had been few house-burnings in east

Cork or west Waterford in 1919–22. Guerrilla war was far more intense in West Cork where the British Army burned down cottages and Tom Barry, the ferocious commander of the local IRA, was torching Anglo-Irish mansions in retaliation. Soldiers set light to the centre of Cork city. The house where my mother was born at Rosscarbery on the coast of West Cork – her parents did not move permanently into Myrtle Grove until the death of Lady Blake in 1926 – was burned to the ground. It was much quieter along the Blackwater. The only mansion to be destroyed in the valley was Cappoquin House, owned by Sir John Keane, and then only because he supported the Free State against the Republicans during the civil war. It was rebuilt by the Irish government ten years later and its Georgian grandeur restored to exactly what it had been. The Keanes, good at sniffing the political breeze, had previously put their furniture into storage and taken casts of the elegant mouldings on the ceiling.

At the time my mother was growing up in Youghal thirty years earlier the Protestants were shocked and frightened by the departure of the English garrison and the establishment of the Irish Free State. They had, after all, stridently justified their opposition to Home Rule by claiming it was the equivalent to Rome rule, which in turn meant the persecution of non-Catholics. In the decade after the Treaty of 1921 a third of all Protestants outside Northern Ireland fled the country. But over the years the Anglo-Irish had become used to their diminished status.[1] Memories of the Protestant Ascendancy had faded (though even when I was about thirteen and in school in Scotland and people asked me where I was from I would say: 'I am ex-Ascendancy,' somehow supposing this would mean something to them). The generation I grew up with were no longer large landowners renting out land to tenant farmers. They did not think much about politics and when they did they were instinctively careful about what they said. We considered visitors from England who spoke in loud voices about the failings of Ireland and the Irish, as naive and ignorant of the new realities. It was not that the local gentry were politically astute, but they had acquired a habit of wariness and caution which Sir Thomas Osborne and Sir Henry Blake would not have recognised.

The Anglo-Irish gentry had never been solely dependent on their position as colonial landowners. Many families, like the Blakes, owned little or no land and, even when they did, this only took care of the eldest son who inherited the property through primogeniture. Younger brothers had to fend for themselves. The options were limited. There were fewer careers available in business, the law, medicine or the Church than in England. The Protestant gentry became far more dependent than their English equivalents on military careers. Since the Duke of Wellington an extraordinarily high proportion of the officer corps in the British Army were Irish Protestants. In the Second World War Bernard Montgomery, Alan Brooke and Harold Alexander were all Anglo-Irish or had Anglo-Irish connections. Field Marshal Frederick Roberts, subject of Kipling's poem 'Bobs', came from south Tipperary and Waterford. Once I came across a faded copy of his memoirs in the library in Myrtle Grove with critical and highly informed comments neatly written in the margin by some fellow Anglo-Irish officer. Sir John Keane of Cappoquin House further up the Blackwater had fought his way from Kandahar to Kabul in Afghanistan in 1839 before being replaced by a less competent general whose regiments were later slaughtered in the Kabul Gorge. As a child I liked a screen in the house at Cappoquin which had paintings of Afghan tribesmen with their long rifles creeping from crag to crag as they sniped at the British redcoats. General Reginald Dyer, the infamous perpetrator of the Amritsar Massacre in 1919, when he ordered his men to fire point-blank into a protest rally, killing 379 demonstrators, came from Castlemartyr, ten miles west of Youghal.

There was nothing particularly surprising in this. Imperial armies in Europe have always recruited from impoverished and reactionary rural gentry. But by the 1950s the British Empire was in terminal decline. The British armed forces were rapidly contracting in size. At the time I was catching polio in 1956 the other big news in the Irish papers was the Suez crisis and the failure of the Anglo-French invasion to overthrow Nasser. The Anglo-Irish lost their old role in the imperial gendarmerie.

Most of my mother's friends lived along the wooded banks of the Blackwater river which runs east through County Cork before entering County Waterford with the dark folds of the Knockmealdown mountains, covered in rhododendron, gorse and bracken, which rise to the north. At the stone bridge at Cappoquin the river turns south and becomes broad and tidal, with reed beds around the mouths of streams flowing into it, until you reach the sea at Youghal. The river, black, pearl-grey and blue depending on the time of day and the light, reflects the green of the trees and is extraordinarily beautiful. The Anglo-Irish had lived in large numbers beside the

Blackwater since the seventeenth century, residing first in semi-fortified manor houses and later in Georgian mansions. The Irish population had also been high before the Famine. Everywhere there were the ruins of cottages. At an early age I liked looking at maps which showed black dots crossing the river. These marked the spots where ferries had once taken people across the Blackwater from jetties and villages that were now just piles of stones.

Our friends lived north–south along the Blackwater rather than east–west along the main road between Waterford and Cork. The only person I remember staying with near Cork city was Penelope Hilliard, who owned Blarney Castle and lived next door to it in an ugly nineteenth-century folly. She owned an enormous but nervous Irish wolfhound who was apt to misinterpret any attempt to pat him on the head as unprovoked aggression and sink his teeth into the extended hand of an unwary guest. When content he would wag his tail which, because of his great size, was about table height and, swinging backwards and forwards, would send cups of tea and glasses of sherry flying across the room. I had seen enough of Irish medieval keeps not to be much interested in the old castle where the Blarney Stone was set into the wall below the ramparts. But I liked a dark cave in the cliff below the castle and a 'Druid' wood with great trees between which a Gothic fantasy of stone circles and huts had been built.

Waterford city was the furthest east we ever travelled to see friends and then infrequently since the only person my mother knew well in the city was Veronica Anderson. The Andersons were descended from both Protestant and Catholic families. Mixed marriages were more frequent in Ireland until Pope Pius IX, a liberal turned reactionary by the 1848 revolution, declared that all children of such a marriage must be brought up as Catholics. Previously the sons of a mixed marriage were brought up in their father's religion and the daughters in their mother's. The Roman Catholic side of the Anderson family was called O'Gorman, originally from Clare, and had produced a number of nationalist notables since the United Irishmen in the 1790s and Daniel O'Connell's campaign for Catholic Emancipation. It was Purcell O'Gorman, a Home Ruler and later a strong supporter of Parnell, who had ended my great-great-grandfather Bernal Osborne's political career by defeating him as MP for Waterford in 1874. O'Gorman's other claim to fame is that, at the time, he was, weighing in at twenty-one stone, the fattest man ever to sit in the House of Commons. He had to have a special niche carved out of his dining-room table so he could reach his food. Veronica's two sons, Benedict and Perry, who were older than me and whom I did not know until much later, were the only Anglo-Irish of the post-Second World War generation in our neighbourhood as radical in politics as my own family.[2]

The incomes of most of the Anglo-Irish had shrunk alarmingly compared to their ancestors'. Having lost their great estates they were dependent on directly farming their land, which brought in little money. On the other hand they did not need very much because food was cheap in Ireland. After the Second World War they could still afford several servants at a time when the English county gentry and upper-middle class were complaining loudly at having, for the first time, to wash their own dishes and clothes. In the same period as my stoutly radical parents were rebuilding Brook Lodge in the late 1940s there was a trickle of arrivals from Britain seeking to escape the recently elected Labour Party. These were known locally as 'the retreat from Moscow' and were the object of some derision. For many of the Anglo-Irish their existence was not unpleasant though somewhat moribund, but if they did not like it the only alternative for them, as it was for much of the Irish population, was to emigrate.

For a few of the more intelligent Anglo-Irish there was another option. They could write and often they wrote very well. The social and national dislocation of life in Ireland as experienced by the remnants of the Protestant Ascendancy was conducive to literary endeavour. Olivia Manning, novelist of the Balkans and the Middle East during the last war, once remarked that she had 'the usual Anglo-Irish sense of belonging nowhere'. At about the same time as my parents were trying to eradicate the rats at Brook Lodge, the novelist William Trevor was growing up the son of the manager of a bank in Youghal's main street. I have wondered since if his father could have been my own father's bank manager, which might explain a strain of melancholy in his son's writing about Ireland. Six miles away, in a white house with a red roof overlooking Ardmore Bay, Molly Keane, successful in writing novels about the Anglo-Irish before the war, was living with her two daughters Sally and Virginia, both with blazing red hair. They came constantly to Brook Lodge. Early in 1956 Ann Pratt, who had been looking after our horses, left us to teach Virginia, who was slowly recovering from pneumonia, how to ride. Virginia recalls that Ann had a furious row with Molly after she went back to Brook Lodge some months later to pick up some clothes, despite the fact that it was known by then that Andrew and I were in hospital with polio.[3] Molly, always a hypochondriac though in this case her fears were sensible, was the only one of our neighbours who blamed my father for constantly travelling backwards and forwards between Ireland and England at the height of the epidemic.

The one novelist specialising in Anglo-Irish themes with whom I found it easy to identify was J. G. Farrell, whose career was cut short when he was swept off a rock by a wave during a storm while fishing in Bantry Bay in West Cork in 1979. This is partly because I enjoyed his account of the Hotel Majestic, the stereotypical Anglo-Irish Big House beset by guerrillas, overabundant foliage and financial ruin, during the War of Independence (the description is in fact based on a hotel Farrell had seen in Rhode Island).[4] But I felt an empathy with Farrell because he caught polio while a student at Oxford two months after I did and was only saved by being rapidly placed in an iron lung. Farrell wrote a grim and telling novel, *The Lung*, about his experience. He describes in terrifying detail how, as he lay in bed in hospital, the virus slowly affected his larynx so he could neither speak nor swallow. He wrote: 'It meant that an army of viruses was now ... marching on the nerve centres of his spinal column. He saw huge ant-like creatures ... crunching away with bared teeth on succulent nerves.'

When my father first came to Youghal he was immediately attracted – a liking which never died – to this 'beautiful, gnarled town where history smells as strong as blood'.[5] Everywhere the squat fortified towers, the homes of the original settlers, stood beside elegant Georgian mansions which had replaced them during more pacific times. The Anglo-Irish houses were concentrated in the valleys. There were few in the damp hills behind Brook Lodge. There were also, after a century of emigration, few enough people of any description. There were more ruined than occupied houses. Three miles beyond our house there was Cornaveigh wood, containing the remains of a village, the outline of the stone walls of its ruined houses blurred by the briars and bushes growing out of them. My mother told me the villagers had been overeager participants in the 1798 uprising and, wrongly supposing the rebellion had already started because of the failure of the coach from Dublin to arrive, had revolted too soon and been destroyed by the forces of order. Later the village acquired the reputation of being haunted because at night passers-by heard groaning sounds coming from the ruins. The real explanation for the ghostly noises, so my mother said, was that survivors would secretly creep back to the village under the cover of darkness to use its water mill, the remains of which are still visible, to grind their corn. Even the most modern maps in the 1950s showed villages which by then barely existed, consisting of a church, a pub and a few houses. They were, as one Irish comedian put it a few years later, the 'sort of village where you plug in your razor and the street lights dim'.

I do not remember the atmosphere in the Anglo-Irish houses as being one of melancholy decay. This was in part because everybody drank heavily, mostly spirits. Wine was regarded with some suspicion as being more of a cordial for the elderly and infirm. The Anglo-Irish had acquired the Irish dread of appearing cold or inhospitable. Hunting acted as social cement. High on a rock a few miles upriver from Ballynatray was Dromana, the house of the Villiers-Stuarts, built on the site of the stronghold of the Earls of Desmond, leaders of frequent doomed rebellions in the fifteenth and sixteenth centuries. When I first saw Dromana, it had a ludicrously large circular ballroom with four fireplaces constructed at some high point in the Villiers-Stuart family fortunes. Once, at the age of sixteen, my mother had suffered a crippling hunting accident near Dromana. Her horse, called Cuchullain, failed to jump a stone bank, turned a complete somersault and landed on top of her. She was carried back to the house. The local doctor said she had broken her collarbone. This turned out to be virtually the only bone she had not broken. She lay flat on her back in bed in the vast bedroom for weeks. Asked one day if there was anything which could be done for her, she said: 'I do get tired of looking at the ceiling all day. If only it weren't bright mauve.' The next day workmen invaded her room. She later recalled: 'They covered me and my bed with a large sheet and then made a great many bumping and dragging noises as they brought in ladders and planks.' When the sheet was removed my mother discovered that the ceiling had been repainted in a peculiarly gloomy mustardy-gold, even more offensive than the previous colour, at which she had to stare for further weeks on end.

The Blackwater valley, with its dark waters and green woods, had always been extraordinarily beautiful, seldom more so than in the 1950s. Emigration had emptied the cottages and in abandoned villages like the one in Cornaveigh wood the ruined walls were submerged by trees, bushes and ferns. When I saw the overgrown gardens of Ballynatray and Myrtle Grove, they were more mysterious and romantic by far than I imagine they were when they were tended by half a dozen gardeners in Victorian times. In most of the world in the twentieth century, nature was retreating and people, increasingly numerous and more prosperous, were on the advance. But Ireland had not shared in the prosperity beginning to transform the rest of Western Europe in the decade after the war. New buildings were few. Trees and ferns were returning to places where they had not grown for four hundred years.

People seldom admit the strong connection between natural beauty and the consequences of economic misery or war. The most beautiful scenery I have ever seen was in the Panjshir valley along the flank of the Hindu Kush mountains in Afghanistan. Two decades of war had destroyed the roads, bridges and all traces of modernity. Horses and donkeys replaced cars and trucks. Wrecked Soviet tanks, rusted red by the weather, were used as part of the walls to fence in fields. A few years earlier I had admired the carpets of wild flowers in the deep battle-scarred valleys of south Lebanon where eagles and kites wheeled overhead, all protected from human interference by old minefields scattered across the land. In Europe the lands and abandoned villages south and west of Chernobyl nuclear power station in the Ukraine are returning to primal wilderness, for ever protected from man by terror of nuclear radiation.

The most remarkable aspect of the Anglo-Irish was that they had survived at all. This was not the fate of most settler elites, planted across the world from Algeria to

Zimbabwe when Europe was at the height of its imperial expansion. But then the history of the Anglo-Irish and their relationship to Ireland was eight hundred years old and deeply complicated. In later life I frequently baulked at telling people I was Anglo-Irish, an explanation which required a rapid excursus into Irish history to make clear that I was not half-English, half-Irish but came from the remnants of the Protestant landowning class. After listening to this potted history with growing impatience, a friend once said to me: 'Best never to tell people you are Anglo-Irish or they will think you an even weirder type of Englishman than they thought you were in the first place.'

Nine

At about 2.30 p.m. on 22 June 1922, my mother, eight years old and with long dark hair, was walking with her nanny in London's Eaton Place, just off Eaton Square, close to where her parents, Jack and Olive Arbuthnot, were living in a mansion at 42 Grosvenor Place. She later recalled:

I saw an old gentleman in a black coat standing on the steps of one of the great pillared doorways of the houses there, when another man standing below him on the pavement pulled out a gun and shot him. The old gentleman half-turned round and then slowly collapsed. I wasn't at all frightened, just supremely interested, and stood there watching while the man with the gun and a companion quietly walked away.[1]

The man whom my mother saw shot to death as he walked up the steps of his house at 36 Eaton Place, was Field Marshal Sir Henry Wilson, until recently Chief of the Imperial General Staff, effectively commander of the entire British Army. Other eyewitnesses confirmed what my mother saw. Wilson had got out of a taxi and already had his door keys in his hands as he was repeatedly shot at close range. By one account he feebly tried to draw a ceremonial sword he was wearing, having just unveiled a war memorial at Liverpool Street station. Wilson was a highly political general, an arch-intriguer and one of the most successful of the great brood of Anglo-Irish military officers. Born in County Longford in the Irish midlands, he was committed to keeping Ulster part of the United Kingdom. In 1914 he had helped organise the 'Curragh Mutiny' when British cavalry officers said they would refuse orders to force Ulster to accept Home Rule along with the rest of Ireland. In his diaries Wilson conveys a breezy arrogance and a contempt for politicians whom he always refers to as 'frocks'. Just before he was killed he had resigned from the army, become a Unionist MP for North Down and was military adviser to the new Northern Ireland government at a time when there were fierce pogroms by Protestants against the Catholics in Belfast.

Of any senior British Army officer, Wilson was the most hated by the IRA and Sinn Fein. They denounced him as a symbol of 'Orange imperialism – predatory militarism tipped with the deadly venom of sectarian bigotry'. Michael Collins ordered his assassination. It was carried out by two leaders of the IRA in London, Reginald Dunne and Joseph O'Sullivan, both veteran soldiers who had fought in the war. O'Sullivan was so badly wounded in the fighting that his right leg had been amputated. He was a strange choice as an assassin, though he was a crack shot, since he was unable to run away after killing the field marshal and was arrested along with Dunne a few minutes later.[2]

The fact that my mother had witnessed the assassination profoundly influenced her life. It led to her spending her youth mostly in Ireland with Lady Blake and not with her more conventional parents. After the shooting, Patricia and her nanny returned home to Grosvenor Place where she excitedly told everybody about the murder. They were openly disbelieving. She later remembered: 'I was told, "Patricia, you really must not tell such lies," and my father said, "There, I told you so, the child's mind is full of murder and bloodshed and now she imagines that she sees horrors wherever she goes even in Eaton Square. It all comes from leaving her so long in Ireland."'

Soon afterwards the evening papers arrived with banner headlines announcing that Sir Henry Wilson had been assassinated by the IRA. This made the Arbuthnots even more worried. They read out an account of the assassination to their daughter. One paper claimed the killers had been chased by a heroic milkman who had followed them hurling milk bottles. My mother calmly told her parents that this was untrue and the gunmen had quietly walked away. Her precise recollection of what had happened further upset them. Her father said: 'She is possibly the only witness and is therefore in grave danger. Now, Patricia, you must *never never never* tell anybody about what you have seen. Not anybody, or the most terrible things will happen to you.'

This was never very likely. Jack Arbuthnot, a major in the Scots Guards who married Olive Blake, the daughter of Sir Henry and Lady Edith in Hong Kong in 1903, had once written a jocular little book on life in Ireland before the First World War. It was called *Arms and the Irishman*, and my mother said it offended both rich and poor, 'the rich because he depicted them in an accurate but derisive way with highly recognisable characters, and the poor because they came out as ignorant peasants of the Pat and Mick variety'. He was quite out of his depth as the War of Independence turned into civil war in southern Ireland and sectarian war raged in the north.

The danger to my mother was very slight. The assassination of Wilson had been very public and there were several eyewitnesses, aside from Patricia, including the taxi-driver who dropped off the field marshal at Eaton Place. There was never any doubt that Dunne and O'Sullivan, though they remained silent in prison, had killed him. They had shot and wounded three other men who pursued them as they tried to escape. But as my mother went upstairs to bed that night she heard Jack Arbuthnot say to Olive: 'Now we can never send her back to Ireland. You can't trust a child to keep her mouth shut, and even if she didn't see the faces of the men who shot Wilson, as she says, it would be only too easy to silence her.'

Her father's words horrified my mother. She was not frightened of being shot but she was appalled by the threat that she would not be allowed to return to Ireland. She had been living happily there with her grandmother Lady Blake during the War of Independence in 1919–21. The rest of the family had moved to London because of the violence in Ireland, although Myrtle Grove was never touched, and her elder brothers were at school at Eton. But the Arbuthnots worried about their youngest daughter. They noticed that, though eight years old, she was totally illiterate and spoke with a strong Irish accent.

Jack Arbuthnot in particular thought she was becoming isolated from the rest of the family by staying in Ireland. He felt she was too much under the influence of her eccentric grandmother whom he neither understood nor particularly liked. He would misquote Oscar Wilde, in one of those sniggering little quips which men of his generation found amusing, saying: 'Lady Blake has a great deal of taste, all of it bad.' My mother seldom saw her father: 'He did not have much impact on my young life, being a shadowy figure who came and went like the family ghost.' But the major did have a point that Patricia was growing up cut off from the outside world since, after the death of Sir Henry in 1918, Edith had become more and more of a recluse in Myrtle Grove. She seldom left the house and then only to sit in the pond garden in fine weather.

My mother had been brought to England early in 1922, first going to a day school and later a fashionable school called Heathfield, which her sister Joan, ten years older than herself, had attended. Many years later my mother wrote:

> From the first day I hated my school and hated all the other little girls in it. Due to my lack of education I couldn't understand the lessons. Anti-Irish feeling was at its height and as I spoke with an Irish brogue, at that time, of which my mother was trying desperately to cure me, the other children immediately guessed my national origin, and were as nasty and as hostile as they could be. I in turn became rude and violent.

It was halfway through her first miserable term at Heathfield that my mother saw Wilson assassinated.

Faced with the threat of a permanent stay in England, which by now she disliked intensely, my mother went on hunger strike. She refused to eat or drink anything but water. She apparently got the idea from the famous hunger strike of Terence MacSwiney, the Lord Mayor of Cork, who had recently starved himself to death after a fast of seventy-four days. His death must have been endlessly talked about by the servants at Myrtle Grove. My mother secretly attended a Mass for the repose of his soul. Although very young, she thought, after discarding the idea of running away as impractical, that a hunger strike might save her from a return to Heathfield and her hated fellow pupils. Her parents, after calling in a doctor, capitulated. They may also have become less worried about their daughter being an eyewitness to the murder after Dunne and O'Sullivan were executed. Jack and Olive agreed that Patricia could return to Myrtle Grove, instead of going back to Heathfield for the autumn term. Their one condition was that she must go with a governess and promise to work hard at her lessons for at least five hours a day.

Finding a governess brave or poor enough to go to Ireland in the middle of a civil war was difficult, but finally a Miss Warwick was employed to teach my mother. At this moment the attention of the Arbuthnots was diverted by another family crisis. Their second-oldest son Terry announced that he wanted to leave Eton early and join the Royal Air Force which had recently been formed out of the old Royal Flying Corps. It was not a popular idea with his parents. They considered it, quite rightly, as being extremely dangerous. They also thought the RAF was not a suitable job for a gentleman and felt that, if any of their sons was to choose a military career, he should join the Navy, the Brigade of Guards or one of a few other select regiments such as the Black Watch. While my mother disappeared to Ireland with Miss Warwick, Terry left Eton for Cranwell Training College to learn how to fly. Having done so he then triumphantly flew a plane over Eton and dropped a message addressed to his brother Bernard, the success of his fine gesture being then somewhat undermined when he crashed the aircraft while trying to land it.[3]

In Myrtle Grove my mother learned how to read and write. There were few modern books in the house and most dated from the eighteenth or nineteenth centuries. She read all twelve volumes of Edward Gibbon's *Decline and Fall of the Roman Empire* by the light of a candle because there was no electricity in the house until years later. Lessons took place in the nursery wing, where Shirley and I were later to play, between 9 a.m. and 1 p.m. with a break at 11 a.m. so my mother could run across the front gravel to have a slice of Madeira cake and a glass of port with her grandmother. Miss Warwick was scandalised by a child being given alcohol, but Lady Blake was adamant that her granddaughter was anaemic and needed building up. As soon as lessons were over my mother spent the rest of the day riding, at first having to make do with three ageing ponies. Only after many pleading letters to her parents in London did they buy her a steady elderly chestnut mare called Isabella, with the promise that she could go hunting as soon as she was twelve.

It must have been a strange life for my mother. Lady Blake, still looking regal and with her long white hair worn high on her head, discouraged visitors with the same excuse she had used for so long in the colonies, that she was not well. She did vary this rule occasionally because, surprisingly enough given that she was by nature an eighteenth-century rationalist, she had become interested in spiritualism. This was flourishing in the years after the First World War. At the other end of County Cork, in Castletownshend, Edith Somerville, author of *Memoirs of an Irish R.M.*, had even formed a unique literary partnership with the departed, producing books supposedly written by 'Somerville and Ross', though Violet Martin, the original Ross, had long since died. Nevertheless, Somerville believed that the ghost of Martin was guiding her pen. A Miss Barlow was invited to stay in Myrtle Grove. She specialised in automatic writing from beyond the grave and she claimed to be able to put Lady Blake in contact with Sir Henry.

At the age of seventeen my mother received a general warning from Olive Arbuthnot about the pitfalls she might expect in the life ahead. At the high point of the briefing her mother said:

And when you marry and have a place of your own, remember above all it's disastrous to let your head gardener *show*. If you do, he'll devote the whole place to getting winners at the county agricultural show or whatever it is. You'll never get so much as a strawberry or hyacinth or stick of asparagus for yourself when you want it.[4]

My father liked this story in which Mrs Arbuthnot appeared, like a character out of P. G. Wodehouse, unable, even in 1931, to foresee a world in which the egocentric ambitions of head gardeners were unlikely to be the main worry in life. But in fact the Arbuthnots were in a good position to ignore economic depression and political turmoil. Unlike most of the Anglo-Irish, they were rich because their family were major shareholders in the Arbuthnot–Latham merchant bank. Jack Arbuthnot, though he had Anglo-Irish and Scottish connections, thought of himself as English and was brought up largely at his father's house at Norton Court in Gloucestershire. My mother, who was never close to him, thought 'he was a most unusual man, certainly not cut out to be a soldier'. He was a good amateur painter and sculptor. He was also a journalist and talented cartoonist, jobs he combined uneasily with his military career. He wrote the original 'Beachcomber' column, a mixture of satire and gossip, for the *Daily Express*, and from 1912 worked for the *Morning Post*. The inevitable clash between performing his military duties and meeting deadlines on the *Express* led to problems unusual for a journalist. On occasion he would have to dash off his column for the *Express* in Fleet Street and then rush across the Thames to Waterloo station where he had ordered a special train to take him to Windsor Castle where he was on guard duty.

The ability to charter special trains argues a large private income, but it had not always been so. He spent heavily. My father, who must have asked him how he first came to work for the *Daily Express*, believed that 'shortly before the death of a relative who later left him a quarter of a million, but was taking some time about it, he found himself rather pressed for money'. He started working part-time as a journalist. My father liked him as 'the genuine kind of High Tory who believes that orders and regulations and forms in triplicate are probably all very well for keeping the machine running and preventing other people from getting out of hand, but should be ignored by people like himself if they happen to interfere in any way with what seems to him good to do at the time'. Called out of the reserves at the start of the First World War, he fought in Somalia and Egypt. At Myrtle Grove a strange relic is preserved of the major's time on the Western Front. On Christmas Day 1914 he collected broken medieval glass from the east window of the cathedral at Ypres, which had been destroyed by shellfire, and reworked the fragments of brown, red, green and clear glass into a cross. He was on duty in the Tower of London when Sir Roger Casement, captured after arriving in Ireland in a German submarine, was incarcerated there before his execution in 1916. The major busied himself finding a new suit of clothes for Casement, regularly broke regulations by letting in his relatives to see him, and made a sketch of him which used to hang in the library in Myrtle Grove.

Olive Arbuthnot died when I was three. I have only a dim recollection of her when she took Shirley and myself on the disastrous expedition to the beach at Goat Island – possibly the memory has stuck because it is the first time I can remember being in a car. She was, by my mother's account, strong-willed, intelligent, interested in the world around her but highly conventional. She was not, however, without a spirit of adventure, was contemptuous of personal discomfort and liked to travel. She married Jack Arbuthnot, an ADC to her father then in his last year as Governor of Hong Kong, in 1903. It was a regal affair and her new husband, liking his creature comforts, had expected that the honeymoon would take place in some luxury hotel. Instead Olive insisted that they should travel to a remote Buddhist monastery in Japan of which she had read. When they arrived he discovered that they would have to sleep on the floor on straw mats. They also found that the monastery was overrun by a large number of rats. Olive later told my mother: 'You know, Daddy didn't like it a bit. He had to stay awake all night shooting at them with his revolver.'

On the death of Lady Blake in April 1926, Olive Arbuthnot became the owner of Myrtle Grove. She and the major spent more time in Ireland. They should have seen more of Patricia, but they had promised her she could go hunting when she was twelve years old. She recorded later that after her twelfth birthday in March she waited with extreme impatience, comparing herself to Jorrocks, the quintessential hunting man created by Surtees, for the moment in November when she could cry: 'Hurrah, hurrah, the dahlias are dead!' It was in November, after the first frosts had blackened the dahlias, that there were the first meets of the two packs my mother was to ride with, the West Waterford and the Mount Uniacke Harriers (in Ireland harriers hunt foxes, not hares). For the next four months she would hunt once a week with each pack until the end of hunting season on or about St Patrick's Day on 17 March.

The hunting was fast because in our part of Ireland at this time there were few ploughed fields and the land was mostly pasture. The main danger was jumping the banks, often as solid as military fortifications and with wide ditches on either side. Hunting was physically taxing since my mother, accompanied by a groom called Willy Brown, often had to ride thirteen miles to a meet in the morning and the same distance back in the evening. This was on top of four or five hours hunting in between. Her social life revolved around hunting. More democratic than in England, it was the one occasion when the Anglo-Irish gentry, the Irish farmers, professional people from the towns and a few newly arrived emigrants from England – though these were few enough in the twenties – met in conditions of some equality.

My mother spent most of the next four years hunting. She saw little of the rest of her family. Her sister Joan loathed anything to do with horses. Aside from the armed services, her four brothers, all with comfortable private incomes, do not seem to have known what to do with themselves. Terry had joined the RAF and Bernard, after Eton, the Royal Navy, where his career was interrupted by one strange incident. Discovering corruption at a naval base in the Far East he denounced those responsible who promptly struck back by locking him up in a mental asylum. Fortunately for Bernard, his mother knew many admirals from her time in Hong Kong and rushed to the Admiralty to get him released. He left the navy in 1938 to join Arbuthnot–Latham, but was almost immediately recalled on the outbreak of war. Terry was at one stage commander of the British air base at Basra in southern Iraq, a place I was to get to know well seventy years later. My mother's eldest brother David never really found a role for himself, though he seems to have liked travelling and there are scattered clippings of articles in family scrap-books describing visits to Poland and the Ukraine in the 1920s. He finally moved to South Africa. My mother's favourite brother, nicknamed Teeny, the member of her family to whom she was closest, also found it difficult to settle into a job until he joined the army in 1939. His mother had confusingly christened him Myles Henry but registered him as Richard Henry, with the result that the army at one moment thought it was employing two offi-cers, both called Arbuthnot. Teeny became a colonel in signals in the Eighth Army and died of malaria in Bari in 1943.

My mother's full-time hunting career came to an end with that accident near Dromana. Her injuries turned out to be far worse than they at first appeared. She lay in bed for weeks. It was only when her mother returned to Ireland from South America, where she had followed Joan during her pursuit of gold in British Guiana, that Patricia was taken to the Bon Secours hospital in Cork. The broken bones had all now set in the wrong position, so they had to be re-broken and reset.

On leaving hospital, she returned to Myrtle Grove and was faced with a long wet Irish winter during which she was forbidden to hunt. The Osbornes and the Blakes always had a taste for prolonged travel abroad as the best way to recover from any crisis. In this case the Arbuthnots thought Patricia would recover more easily if she went to Biskra, a town they had visited on the edge of the Sahara in southern Algeria. Aged only sixteen, she was accompanied by a maid called Sheelagh who had never been out of Ireland before and was initially terrified of foreigners. The Arbuthnots gave my mother a list of people they knew in Biskra. She almost immediately met the one person they had deliberately not included, Clare Sheridan, a sculptress and courtesan, whose lovers had included everybody from Trotsky to Charlie Chaplin. She told my mother that Trotsky, whose head she was sculpting, had loaded her with sables and other gifts 'to the extreme annoyance of the then Mrs Trotsky who, Clare told me, once publicly slapped her face'. To Clare's distress the sables and other gifts were confiscated by border guards as she left the Soviet Union.

It must have been shortly after my mother's return from Algeria that Olive Arbuthnot warned her about the danger of allowing your head gardener to become obsessed with the local agricultural show. But the head gardener question could hardly arise until after marriage and to this end they needed to present Patricia at court and 'bring her out' as a debutante. My mother was impatient in later years when former debutantes were retrospectively critical of these bizarre upper-class rituals, soon to disappear in the turmoil of war, or saw them through a haze of nostalgia. She said: 'I personally had a very good time and found all the ramifications of the labyrinthine etiquette interesting and amusing.' Her presentation at court took place in the summer of 1931. A photograph taken at the time shows my mother in a full white evening dress with a two-foot train and long white kid gloves extending above the elbow. Just visible on her head are three white ostrich feathers and eighteen inches of white tulle falling behind her neck. In her hand is a long ostrich-feather fan.

By tradition debutantes and their families waited for two hours in chauffeur-driven black limousines, the queue stretching down the Mall, until they were admitted to

Buckingham Palace at 8 p.m. Given that this was the height of the Depression, Patricia was subsequently surprised that the crowds were not hostile. More than half a century later my mother recalled the long wait on the Mall:

> Inside our car we were having a rather uncomfortable time. Both my parents were in a vile temper, my father because he was wearing the dress uniform of a major of the Scots Guards and he hadn't bought a new uniform since his retirement from the army, so the tunic was extremely tight. It was also hot and stuffy in the car with the windows on the pavement side shut. My mother was annoyed because Daddy had announced earlier that as we should not get supper in Buckingham Palace until after the last debutante had been presented, he would get hungry – so he had brought sandwiches which, as he had nowhere else to put them, he had put in his bearskin helmet ... Due to the heat, the lavish amount of butter in the sandwiches had melted, soaking his bearskin, and was spreading everywhere. Mummy was terrified it would get on her, or my, dress. There she sat in her diamond tiara, trying to look calm and benign and muttering under her breath: 'Jack, Jack, how *could* you, I shall never forgive you.'[5]

At the age of nineteen, two years after coming out as a debutante, my mother married a Lloyd's underwriter called Arthur Byron. When I was in my late teens she would use her experience as a signal warning against early marriage. She and her new husband had gone to Sicily for the honeymoon. It was there, she would say, 'while walking with Arthur on a beach near Palermo I thought to myself, "I've married the *most boring* man in the world."' In her autobiography she is kinder, commenting only that she and Arthur had 'really very little in common beyond physical attraction and a mutual desire to have a good time'. Her father, the major, had been delighted that his daughter had chosen somebody quite so conventional – and fairly well off – to marry. She said: 'I had sometimes seen my father look at me warily, like someone who owns a strange pet whose temper they are not quite sure of, and I felt he was relieved that at last I appeared to be doing something sensible.'

Her mother had more misgivings believing her daughter was too young to settle down. She told her:

> I don't think you should marry an Englishman. I am quite sure that when you have seen enough of the world, you will go back to Ireland and he won't like to live there permanently. Englishmen seldom do. You will also slide back into your old ways with your friends in Ireland, and make him feel an outsider. Of course it is your decision, and as your father approves I will make no objection, but think it over very carefully.

As a result of her mother's doubts the marriage was delayed well into 1933 when it took place on a grand scale in St Mark's in North Audley Street.

My mother, though not particularly political, could see the world was becoming more dangerous, and if she and Arthur wanted to travel they should do so immediately.

They were not short of money. Arthur, aside from his income from Lloyd's, had inherited a large sum of money for a curious reason. It came from his grandfather who had owned a country house and large estate in Purley, later a suburb of London but in the mid-nineteenth century the depths of the country. He kept a pack of hounds but was frustrated because, as London expanded, he found that the only covers he could draw were increasingly his own. As houses sprouted around his estate the grandfather furiously rejected increasingly remunerative offers to buy his land. He lived to be very old, his children were forced to emigrate to make a living, but he refused to sell an inch of the estate, now a green island in the London sprawl. As soon as he died the executors sold the land for a large sum which was inherited by Arthur.

Soon after their return from Sicily the Byrons started on a year-long tour of the world. They travelled west through the US, Canada and, after six months in Tahiti, on to Malaya and Siam as it then was. Patricia had been asked by Admiral Sir William Goodenough, the head of the Royal Geographic Society, to investigate nomadic tribes in northern Siam. She was struck by the extreme racism of British colonial society. Once in Malaya, arriving at a local English club with flowers in her hair, she was told by the wife of some planter: 'You must take those flowers out of your hair immediately. Only native women wear flowers in their hair.' Disgusted by their narrow prejudices, my mother reflected how right her grandmother had been, as the wife of the governor, to feign illness 'as an excuse not to have to entertain the wives of the English colonials'. Travelling on to Ceylon where her family owned a profitable tea estate, purchased by Sir

Henry Blake, she began to feel increasing exasperation at the evident poverty of the Sinhalese villagers, despite the rich fertility of the land.

Back in London Patricia gave birth to a son called Darell. She was never very interested in babies. She came into her own as soon as children could engage in practical activities such as building dams or tree houses. She once again felt bored in London and quarrelled with her nanny who wanted the Byron crest painted in miniature on both sides of the pram. My mother pointed out that the crest was of a mermaid, whose naked breasts already caused ribald comment when engraved on silver spoons and forks. Arthur returned to Lloyd's. Patricia and her brother Teeny had meanwhile made friends with people more liberal and intellectual than they had been brought up to know. Patricia was obviously restless. At this point Admiral Goodenough telephoned her to ask if she would like to make a language map of tribes in Central Africa. It was an ambitious plan for a twenty-two-year-old girl since Goodenough wanted her to start in Kampala in Uganda, visit Rwanda, travel west through the forests down the River Congo and continue through the French Equatorial Africa. They were then to travel north-west, ending up at Lake Chad, and return across the Sahara. Olive Arbuthnot, who did like small babies, offered to look after Darell while my mother was away.

It was an extraordinary journey and one I was familiar with from an early age because my mother was a good photographer. On her earlier travels to the Far East she had taken pictures of the temples of Angkor Wat, Cambodia, Siam and Ceylon. In Central Africa she took photographs of people, villages and animals wherever she went. When I was very young the photographs were kept loose in a large drawer of a Regency desk in Brook Lodge – for some reason they were never put in a scrapbook – and from about the age of four I used to look with fascination at pictures of pygmies in the Belgian Congo, witch-doctors, mud villages, Watusi dancers and elephants with their vast ears and long tusks. Other boys brought up before the final decline of the British Empire would later record the profound influence on them of John Buchan's *Greenmantle* or Rider Haggard's *King Solomon's Mines*. But in my case these books merely confirmed the early impression created by my mother's pictures that the rest of the world was an exciting place full of adventures to be visited as soon as possible.

My mother returned to England in the autumn of 1938 to find that the rest of her family had gone to Ireland. A few days later she received a telephone call from her mother saying that Darell was very ill. He had fallen in the garden at Myrtle Grove and scratched his nose. The graze turned septic and the doctors said he had blood poisoning. He was taken to the Bon Secours hospital in Cork where Patricia had lain in bed for months after her hunting accident eight years before. A few years later and Darell could have been saved by antibiotics, but by the time my mother arrived in Cork the doctors thought there was little chance of him surviving. Patricia wrote:

He lay in his little white cot, semi-conscious, Thank God at least he was not suffering. I sat by him watching his life slowly ebb away. I was frozen with despair and guilt. I had seen so little of him in his short life: I should never have left him . . . In Africa

I had been so busy and interested in the new places and people I was seeing that I had hardly given a thought to those at home.

I became conscious of Darell's existence quite early because I was given his christening mug, a pretty silver goblet with 'Darell Byron from Beatrix St Albans' engraved on it. I was a little resentful as to what his name was doing on my mug, and curious about his existence or lack of it.

Back in London my mother fell into a deep depression. Her family was initially sympathetic and then by turns impatient and irritated, suggesting that she pull herself together. She eventually thought she might have contracted some disease in Africa and went to the Institute of Tropical Medicine where they showed great interest in her case, but only, she discovered, because they wanted to find out why she had never got malaria. The death of Darell also convinced her to decide, she later told me, that her marriage to Arthur Byron was coming to an end. She came to the conclusion that she ought to leave London and travelled to Ruthenia in the far west of Czechoslovakia to write articles for the *Evening Standard*. On her return Arthur volunteered for the army and she joined the ARP, the Air Raid Precautions organisation, and went to work in a deep bunker under Praed Street in Paddington. At about the same time she went to a party at Arlington House, just below the Ritz, given by a rich American woman called Connie Bainbridge where she met Claud Cockburn, notorious as the communist editor of his newsletter the *Week*. He asked to be introduced to her because he had read her articles about Ruthenia, a place he knew and loved from the time he lived in Central Europe.

Some months later she told her parents that she was going to leave Arthur for my father. They reacted with bewildered fury. In a final angry meeting before disinheriting her, Jack Arbuthnot, embarrassed and red-faced, ran through the reasons why he opposed the marriage. He concluded by saying: 'Don't you realise, Patricia, that if you go ahead with this mad plan you will never be allowed into the Royal Enclosure at Ascot ever again?' He had another quibble. He was proud that he held a certain record at the Carlton Club. Three of his sons and his son-in-law were all members. Now, though Arthur Byron would presumably remain a member, he would no longer be the major's son-in-law and the record would be lost.

Olive Arbuthnot – much to the delight of my father who had never expected to hear the phrase actually used – called Claud 'a traitor to his class'. She too sought to dissuade my mother from running away with a penniless Red, whom she probably suspected of being after her daughter's money. 'Do you realise that, if your brothers were in the diplomatic service, a scandal of this kind would force them to resign?' she said.

'But they are not in the diplomatic service,' my mother replied, not unreasonably.

'That,' said Mrs Arbuthnot, impatiently hammering the floor with her walking stick, 'is not the point.'

My mother was distressed by the reaction of her parents, of whom she was extremely fond; more practically, for the first time in her life, she was seriously short of money. But she was not entirely surprised. 'I doubt if any English family of the same class would have made such a fuss,' she reflected later. 'In the old Anglo-Irish culture marriages were not just the business of the parties most nearly concerned. They were family matters involving settlements and legal contracts. It was, after all, only one or two generations since arranged marriages had been the rule rather than the exception.'

The breach between my parents and the Arbuthnots did not last very long. The war gave them other things to think about. By the end of 1940, as German aircraft bombed London, my mother was working in the ARP headquarters controlling the dispatch of fire brigades, ambulances and rescue equipment. Three of her brothers were in the navy, army and air force respectively. Major Arbuthnot's pride in his record family membership of the Carlton Club must have seemed less relevant when it was destroyed by a German bomb. He painted a colourful little cartoon of its members creeping on their hands and knees towards the door as the bombs got closer.

In 1944 my parents' house in St John's Wood was destroyed by a V-1 rocket. Neither of them was at home. Patricia sent a brief telegram from Brampton in Cumberland to her mother in London which illustrates her swift practicality in dealing with disaster. It reads:

HOPE YOU ARE ALRIGHT MY HOUSE DESTROYED COULD YOU CONTACT CLAUDS SECRETARY MRS RISNER CHANCERY 6565 ABOUT SAVING REMAINS OF FURNI- TURE AND STORING WILL TRY AND RING YOU TONIGHT MY NUMBER BRAMPTON 137 LOVE PATRICIA.

She does not bother to mention the destruction of the house in her autobiography. Claud, equally typically, devotes three lines to the destruction of the house and two pages to the effect it had on a favourite cat which had previously worshipped him and seen him as the provider of all good things. Not illogically the cat blamed him for the bomb which had destroyed her world. Whenever he approached she fled shrieking into the garden where she hid until he had departed.

Ten

My father once said that the report that God was on the side of the big battalions was propaganda put about by big battalion commanders to demoralise their opponents. He saw the rich and powerful as highly vulnerable to journalistic guerrilla warfare of a type largely invented by himself. Just before he died in 1981 Graham Greene wrote of him: 'If I were asked who are the two greatest journalists of the twentieth century, my answer would be G. K. Chesterton and Claud Cockburn . . . Perhaps Claud Cockburn will prove to be more influential, for he discovered the influence that can be wielded by a mimeo-graphed news-sheet.' This was the *Week*, the radical newsletter he started with a capital of forty pounds in 1933 after resigning from his job as the New York correspondent of *The Times*.

It seemed a propitious moment. Britain was still gripped by the Depression and Hitler had just taken power in Germany. My father supposed that many intelligent people understood that the mainline press presented a sanitised and misleading version of the increasingly tumultuous world in which they lived. This may well have been so, but at first they were depressingly slow to embrace the alternative view of events presented by the *Week*. Its survival looked doubtful until it was unexpectedly saved by Ramsay MacDonald, then prime minister, who, stung by criticism, roundly denounced the hitherto obscure newsletter at a press conference in the Geological Museum in South Kensington.

My father wrote a fine description of the circumstances in which MacDonald had attacked him. The prime minister, leader since 1929 first of a Labour government and then of one dominated by the Conservatives, was hosting a World Economic Conference, an event from which he alone believed some good might come. Although the conference was visibly dead on its feet, the press had politely said that 'useful spadework' was being done. The *Week* commented acidly that the only spade it could detect at work at the conference was that of the gravediggers. My father reported:

Mr MacDonald came down to the Conference looking, as someone remarked, as though he were on his way to Clarkson's to hire a crown of thorns. He convened a special off-the-record press conference in the crypt. He said he had a private warning to utter. Foreign and diplomatic correspondents from all over the world jostled past mementoes of the Ice Age to hear him. For as a warning utterer he was really tip-top. In his unique style, suggestive of soup being brewed on a foggy Sunday evening in the West Highlands, he said that what we saw on every hand was plotting and conspiracy . . . and here in his hand was a case in point. Everyone pushed and stared, and what he had in his hand was that issue of the *Week*; and he went on to quote from it, and to warn one and all to pay no heed to the false prophets of disaster. This was good strong stuff and stimulating to these people who hitherto had never heard of the *Week* and, but for this, possibly never would have.[1]

The idea behind the *Week* was simple enough. My father was struck by the contrast between the colourful information passing between politicians, diplomats, bankers and newspapermen at their gatherings and the 'tight-lipped drabness' of the newspapers being sold in the street outside. He thought that there must be enough people, deeply dissatisfied by what they were reading, to form a potential pool of enthusiastic readers. While living in Germany and the US he became aware of a little-noticed but potent and above all cheap means of reaching this audience. The power of mass-produced newspapers, the radio and the cinema to mould public opinion was obviously enormous. All required a great deal of money to establish and run. Those who dissented from the views expressed in the conventional media often despaired of effectively counter-attacking the powers that be. My father believed they were too pessimistic. Just before leaving the US in 1932 he had written a book called *High Low Washington 1930–32*. It was an insider's account of Washington produced at some speed during a broiling summer to finance his return to Europe. 'Among technical devices which everyone knows are revolutionising modern government, the humble mimeograph machine is seldom mentioned,' he wrote, adding that it 'is one of the few remaining weapons which still gives small and comparatively poor organisations a sporting chance in a scrap with large and wealthy ones'. A few months later in Berlin he observed with keen interest that General Schleicher, an unsavoury ally of Hitler, distributed a weekly newsletter filled with comment and information, sold only by subscription, which had an influence out of all proportion to its circulation.

The calculations behind founding the *Week*, as explained by my father, sound so convincing that it is surprising that there were not hundreds of newsletters being founded all over Europe and the US in the early 1930s. It was evidently more difficult than it looked. True, it did not take much money to start a newsletter, but most people would have tried to raise more than the forty pounds he borrowed from a friend. An office was rented in an attic on the seventh floor of 34 Victoria Street (now part of the site of Scotland Yard). Even the mimeograph was rented. This overt display of indigence, though all too accurately reflecting dire financial reality, had another purpose. Most people who sue the media in Britain, then as now, do so in order to make money. My father wanted potential litigants, if they or their emissaries ever reached his office by way of an elderly lift and a staircase resembling a stepladder, to be wholly convinced of the poverty of the organisation against whom they were about to bring a legal action.

From the beginning Claud was determined that the *Week* should have a very defined personality. It was never going to look very distinguished but he decided to make a virtue of necessity and ensure it was distinctive by printing it in dark brown ink on buff-coloured paper. 'It was,' he wrote with some pride, 'not merely noticeable, it was unquestionably the nastiest looking bit of work that ever dropped on to a breakfast table.' He thought it a mistake for editors to produce a mosaic of articles in the hope that one or other of them would appeal to the reader. He was convinced that this approach meant that the paper would have no personality with which to repel or appeal to the reader. It was like a fisherman casting a net of impressive extent but with holes in the mesh so big that fish would swim through them. He would say that in producing a paper or magazine it was the wrong approach 'to make everybody like you a bit because you want to make a smaller number like you a lot or at least enough to buy your paper. And if they do not like you at least they will notice you.' Even with a grubby newsletter he was very precise on the impression he wanted to make on the reader. Although it was sent in cheap brown envelopes he insisted that they be sealed in order to increase the sense of confidentiality, despite the fact that this tripled the price of postage.

My father had great confidence in his own judgement, particularly anything to do with newspapers. But even his optimism about the prospects for the *Week* faltered in those first weeks as subscriptions failed to roll in. In the six years before returning to London in 1933 he had lived almost entirely in Germany and the US. He feared he had exaggerated the speed with which readers in Britain would take to the new publication. The new venture suffered from other disadvantages. He had acquired an ageing circulation list of 1,200 names from a temporarily defunct magazine called *Foreign Affairs*. Many turned out to be dead or indifferent. After the first few issues he found that 'the number of paying customers secured by the first

185

circularisation was seven. Just seven.' It was only slowly, aided by assaults such as that from Ramsay MacDonald, that the readers began to subscribe.

My father was the arch-exponent of this type of guerrilla journalism which at its best, and even with surprisingly little resources, can shake the mighty from their seats. Often its proponents are surprised by their ability to intimidate the powerful. I recall once in Haiti a friend who ran a radical Creole radio station telling me that he had received a visit from a particularly ferocious gunman from a Tonton Macoute death squad. He had repeatedly denounced the man's crimes on air. My friend's office was on the top floor of a building in Port-au-Prince in which the final flight of stairs was closed off by a locked metal gate. He was nevertheless extremely nervous as he heard the Macoute rattling the bars of the gate and shouting. He supposed he was being threatened with imminent torture and death, the usual fate of critics of the Haitian regime at this time. My friend only relaxed when he made out that in fact the gunman was yelling: 'I demand an apology' at the top of his voice. 'I suddenly realised that the regime was on its way out,' he said.

Optimistic though he was about the prospects for his newsletter, Claud was nevertheless agreeably surprised by the extent of its success. He boasted that five years after he started it the foreign ministries of eleven nations, all the embassies in London, King Edward VIII and Charlie Chaplin were subscribers: 'Blum read it and Goebbels read it, and a mysterious warlord in China read it. Senator Borah quoted it repeatedly in the American Senate and Herr von Ribbentrop, Hitler's Ambassador in London, on two separate occasions demanded its suppression on the ground that it was the source of all anti-Nazi evil.' He coined the phrase 'the Cliveden Set' to describe the anti-appeasement lobby.

There had been confidential newsletters before but not quite in the style of the *Week*. It 'was an intoxicating newspaper', wrote Cyril Connolly many years later:

> Written for the knowing by those in the know, it was genuinely diabolical in that it never put anything past its opponents. Motive was peeled from motive, betrayal was found under betrayal, bribe upon bribe, and always in the august and persuasive language of *The Times*. I am sure it was his *Times* manner that spared Mr Cockburn a single libel action – not, as he thinks, the poverty of his organisation. His victims literally could not believe their eyes.[2]

Connolly showed a certain simplicity in believing that it was the grandeur of my father's style which deterred litigants rather than the knowledge that they would not make a penny. As editor he also resolutely refused to apologise though he always expressed willingness to publish a follow-up article if whoever was threatening to sue him would provide information showing that the earlier story was baseless. 'It was at this point,' he said, 'that one could usually detect from their expression that the thought passing through their minds was that if their client took their case to court he would probably make a bigger monkey out of himself than he was likely to make out of me.'

Even after almost three-quarters of a century accounts in the *Week* of long-forgotten crises are compelling, the stories convincingly full of names and details. 'Generalities are often boring,' my father would say. 'Details almost never are.' His reputation suffered in later years because he openly and repeatedly declared that he would print rumours as well as facts, arguing that both were frequently of equal significance. Equally open to misunderstanding was what he called 'the factual heresy', the belief that there is a predetermined number of significant facts in the world for which the journalist goes in search:

> To hear people talking about facts you would think that they lay about like pieces of gold ore in the Yukon days waiting to be picked up – arduously, it is true, but still definitely and visibly – by strenuous prospectors whose subsequent problem was only how to get them to market.

He saw this view as misleading though useful to journalists and newspapers who want to claim saint-like objectivity. He said: 'All stories are written backwards – they are supposed to begin with the facts and develop from there, but in reality they begin with a journalist's point of view from which the facts are subsequently organised.' Of course, it has often suited journalists in terms of their own self-esteem to argue that their job is the apolitical pursuit of factual truths. This helpfully diverts the public's attention away from the fact that the point of view from which they write may be determined not by them but by the proprietor of the newspaper for which they write.

All this makes the journalist's job both easier and more difficult than it looks. It is more difficult because even before they come into his possession, facts frequently have a spin to them. Nobody tells you their own or other people's secrets without a reason. This may be love of truth or shock at the misdeeds of their superiors or to divert, but a motive is always there. Again journalists seldom expatiate on why they have been told something. This is partly because, contrary to every Hollywood film ever made about reporters, they are ill-equipped to extract information which others do not want to impart. People do not naturally tell facts which incriminate themselves, or might land them in jail, except under legal duress. Thus the most damaging information about the Watergate burglary published in the *Washington Post*, supposedly a high point in investigative journalism in the twentieth century, was discovered by prosecutors, judges and law-enforcement agencies who then leaked it to the newspaper. A journalist might like to be a spy but generally ends up as a conduit for information. There is, of course, nothing wrong with this so long as the journalists do not mislead the public into thinking they alone are capable of defending their freedoms.

My father's belief that what matters most in a journalist or a publication is the sceptical point of view, his overall political stance, also makes the journalist's job easier. Many facts are secret simply because the press has decided not to publish them. Malcolm Muggeridge and my father, while working on *Punch* in the 1950s, had discussed setting up a magazine free from the commercial pressures and proprietorial control under which they were then working. 'Then the *Eye* came along in answer to their prayers,' writes Richard Ingrams, for many years its editor. 'Claud and Malcolm subsequently acted as godfathers to the fledgling organ.'[3]

189

Even after living in Brook Lodge for fifteen years my father did not lose his enthusiasm or ability to harry the government. In August 1963, thirty years after he had published the first issue of the *Week*, he was guest editor of *Private Eye* at the height of the Profumo scandal. He immediately broke a media convention by revealing that C, the chief of MI6, whose identity was supposedly a secret, was in fact Sir Dick White. He did so in a small paragraph in a column written under his name headed 'Note to foreign agents', saying that Sir Dick was 'the head of what you romantically term the British Secret Service'. When the Cabinet papers were made public in 2000 it emerged that the story had led to panic in Whitehall. Sir Burke Trend, the Cabinet secretary, immediately summoned a meeting but it regretfully decided that it would not prosecute my father because his source was unknown and he was unlikely to disclose it. They also reflected that the identity of C was, in any case, widely known in Fleet Street.

Officials even dragged Harold Macmillan, the prime minister, into the affair, suggesting that C and Sir Roger Hollis, then the head of MI5, should have discreet meetings with 'responsible editors'. (Ironically a cabal in MI5 later came to believe that Sir Roger was a Soviet agent, a prime reason for their suspicion being his friendship with the communist Claud Cockburn at Oxford. My father said he scarcely knew Sir Roger then, though he was an old friend of his brother Christopher Hollis.) In a splendid piece of obfuscation which my father would have enjoyed reading, Sir Burke discussed with fellow Whitehall mandarins the whole issue of secrecy and the media. He wrote: 'It is a matter not so much of concealing as of withholding and what is withheld is not so much the truth as the facts.'[4]

Not that my father entirely lacked caution. A year later he and Peter Cook, editing another issue of *Private Eye*, named the Kray twins as the two East End gangsters who had been terrorising much of London. Their criminal activities were often referred to in the press but they had never previously been identified. The piece, before listing the allegations against the Krays, gingerly stated: 'Either the charges are true, in which case the newspapers should have the guts to publish them, whatever the risk of libel action. Or they are untrue or grossly exaggerated, in which case they should stop scaring people with this horror mob movie of London under terror.' The article ended by noting that the *Eye* was not anxious to be sued for libel, have its kneecaps blown off or be burned as a sort of reluctant Buddhist, and gently warned the reader that this might be the last issue under present management.

The fearless authors evidently took the possibility of retaliation by the Krays quite seriously because Cook speedily retreated to Tenerife and my father as promptly to Ireland. Cook said their motto was 'Publish and be absent'.[5]

My father was born in Peking in 1904, the son of Henry Cockburn, a British diplomat who spent most of his career in China and the Far East. Four years earlier he and his wife had survived the siege of the legation quarter by the Boxers. Once my grandfather watched from the walls as the insurgents derisively displayed the crucified body of a messenger he had tried to send through their lines. The

191

Far East was already being shaken by war and rebellion ten years before Europe was similarly convulsed after 1914. Claud was born on the day the Japanese blew up the Russian flagship *Petropavlovsk* at the height of the Russo-Japanese war.

At the age of two he was sent back to Britain accompanied by a Chinese amah, or nanny, first to England and then to stay with a grandmother in Scotland. The amah was unhappy because boys shouted and threw stones at her on account of her blue trousers. She also feared that she and Claud would be attacked by tigers when they went for walks in the hills. When his parents returned on leave two years later they found their son only spoke Chinese and, in spite of his rage, they sent the amah back to China. Patricia believed he never forgave his mother. He recalled standing up in his bath shouting at her in Chinese, which she did not understand: 'I wish you would go away to a far country.' He later entirely forgot his Chinese though he hoped that, like American litigants suing those responsible for some childhood trauma, he might one day have a shock leading to a total recovery of memory and suddenly be able to speak the language fluently again. One night, just before he died in 1981, he began to speak deliriously about Chinese pirates besieging the house and asked for his mother to tell Number One Houseboy something about firearms.

His father had now moved from Peking to Korea where he was first British minister and then consul general. He was disgusted by the British agreement with the Japanese under which Japan gained complete control of Korea. Offered another post, he announced he was weary of the Foreign Office and resigned in 1908 at the age of forty-nine. It was a slightly surprising end to a career which had also had a surprising beginning. His father, the grandson of Lord Henry Cockburn, the notable judge, historian and liberal leader in Edinburgh during the Scottish Enlightenment, was a judge in India when it was ruled by the East India Company. My grandfather hoped to pursue a similar career by entering the Indian civil service. Highly intelligent and well-educated, he had every hope of passing the examination until he unwisely disclosed to his father that under the influence of German philosophy he had become an atheist. His father, as a former judge in Bombay and a firm believer in Christianity as the cement of the British Empire, rushed to London and by vigorous pulling of strings ensured that his son had no chance of ruling any segment of India. Many years later Claud protested mildly that 'he might at least have tried to convert you'. His father replied:

> But you see, he took it for granted that everybody's views were as unshakeable as his own. And he would have thought, too, that I might be tempted to a false pretence at conversion – which would have been bad for my moral character; and then, later, when I was Lieutenant Governor, I might have come out in my true colours and started massacring the missionaries, or forced them to give readings from Feuerbach from their pulpits.[6]

Regretting, nevertheless, that he had spoken so openly of his religious views, my grandfather sold his books and disappeared from the family home. When next heard of he had sat and passed the exam for the Eastern Consular

Service from which he could pass into the Diplomatic Service in the Far East. By the age of nineteen he was the British vice-consul in Chungking, the isolated Chinese city built into the crumbling cliffs above the Yangtze river. Even after he finally left China he secretly yearned to return. Once, after the family had lived in four or five different houses in southern England in as many years, he explained to my father that 'he had come to the conclusion that it would be really more satisfactory to buy a house in the hills west of Peking, but he wanted to give England every chance'.

The years he lived with his grandmother and his Chinese amah were the only extended period that my father lived in Scotland. Despite this he was always self-consciously Scottish and sent my brothers and myself to school at Glenalmond in Perthshire on the grounds that Scottish education was better than anything available in England (a calculation which was largely correct going by the accounts of English contemporaries). His attachment to Scotland had much to do with his admiration for his great-grandfather, whose witty anecdotal style in *Memorials of his Time* was much like his own. There was also political empathy. An advocate of parliamentary reform, Henry Cockburn was exposed to the violent blast of the Tory reaction in Scotland in the twenty years after the French Revolution. The atmosphere was similar to that in central Europe, where Claud spent so many of his formative years in the decade after the Russian Revolution.

I myself at an early age was more attracted by the activities of Admiral Sir George Cockburn, a highly successful naval commander during the Napoleonic Wars, who burned Washington in 1814 as part of the Anglo-American war. He was an aggressive and successful sea captain who had been ordered to cruise Chesapeake Bay to destroy American shipping and seize horses for the cavalry of a British army being shipped across the Atlantic to America. While engaged in this mission, he made the interesting and potentially remunerative discovery that there were warehouses on the creeks along the Chesapeake stuffed with valuable tobacco. Instead of rounding up cavalry horses, Cockburn and his men spent their time loading plundered tobacco on to their ships. Only at the last moment, perhaps conscious that he had been remiss in his military duties, did the admiral make a successful lunge at Washington where he burned the White House and Congress. He gave particular attention to wrecking the offices of a newspaper which had made rude fun of the way his name was spelled.

Just as the First World War broke out my father's family moved to Berkhamsted so he could attend the nearby public school. It was an experience that, on the whole, he enjoyed. Fortunately for him he was too young to move from the cadet corps into the army before the war ended. But a rise in the cost of living had left his father financially embarrassed. A friend told him there was a job going in an inter-allied financial mission to look after the finances of Hungary. Claud later explained:

My father asked whether the circumstances of his knowing almost nothing about Hungary and absolutely nothing about finances would be a disadvantage. His friend said that was not the point. The point was that they had had a man doing this job who knew all about Hungary and a lot about finance, but he had been seen picking his teeth with a tram-ticket in the lounge of the Hungaria hotel and was regarded as socially impossible. My father said that if such were the situation he would be prepared to take over the job.[7]

Claud became a boarder at Berkhamsted while his parents moved into a large and expensive suite in the Hotel Gellert in Budapest. They expected to stay there only temporarily because part of the purpose of moving to central Europe was to save money by taking advantage of the low cost of living. They looked at many houses over the next three and a half years but in all of them his father detected some serious defect. Claud believed the real problem was that none of them was in the hills west of Peking. His parents never moved out of the Gellert and spent more money than if they had remained in England.

It was a heady political atmosphere for a sixteen-year-old just arrived from an English public school. On Claud's first visit to Budapest the guide from the Gellert, after meeting him on his arrival at the railway station, briefly stopped on the journey to the hotel on a bridge over the Danube. He explained that he wanted to show the young Englishman the exact spot in the water where he had seen bobbing against the piles of the bridge the bodies of three hundred Reds, shot or driven at bayonet point into the river after the crushing of Bela Kun's Communist uprising. Not surprisingly my father soon developed a sense of revulsion, shared by many young men from the victorious powers, for the results of the German defeat. He wrote: 'No doubt this reaction was strongest among people who, like myself, lived in central Europe at the time, and were exposed to the well-organised lamentations of Hungarian landowners, German steel barons in the Ruhr and ulcerated international bankers.' At Berkhamsted he had been a strong Conservative but, viewing the consequences of the war from the windows of the Gellert, he came to see them as a hideous betrayal of the principles for which the war had supposedly been fought. In England John Maynard Keynes and other liberals were already denouncing the Treaty of Versailles as a crime. Claud later thought that it was one of the many grotesque ironies of the era that the great liberal economist was expounding the same ideas as extreme nationalists in central Europe 'who would cheerfully have chopped his ears off had they seen the slightest profit to themselves in doing so'.[8]

It was in Budapest, while drinking iced beer on the terrace of the Hotel Gellert, that my father received a telegram from Keble College, Oxford, asking simply: 'ARE YOU MEMBER CHURCH OF ENGLAND?' He realised that he must have won a scholarship to Keble, then a bastion of the Anglican Church. He was at first dismayed that he might lose the scholarship because of this religious hurdle but was reassured by his father that he had been baptised in the Anglican faith. For the next three years he moved between central Europe and Oxford, a university where he noted that it was still just possible, despite the terrible casualty lists, to imagine that the First World War had not taken place. His philosophy tutor would say of any philosophical idea less than two hundred years old: 'I think you'll find that it's pretty well been exploded.' Once my father thought he had checkmated the tutor by giving him a volume of philosophy just published in Budapest and which he could not possibly have seen. After some hours the tutor returned the volume remarking: 'I rather gather that the man is likely pretty soon to be exploded.'

On leaving Oxford he applied for a travelling fellowship given by Queen's College which would pay him 250 pounds a year for two years to live in a country of his choice. This was an exiguous amount even then but my father believed he knew of places in central Europe where he could live in modest comfort on such a sum. His family was at first dismayed by the plan having hoped, because of the unexpected expense of living in Hungary, that he would move more rapidly into full-time employment. Instead he went to live for some months in an impoverished village in the Cevennes in 1926, where he intended to improve his French, a command of modern languages being essential to winning the fellowship. His German, which he had taught himself at Berkhamsted, was already fluent.

On his return to Oxford for the fellowship interview his main fear was that his creditors would pounce and issue writs before he could win it. Since the fellowship was intended as something of a finishing school for graduates intending to enter respectable professions like the Foreign Office, he was also worried that his evident poverty might lead the examiners to doubt his suitability. When he talked my father liked to cross one leg over the other and gesticulate with his hands. But he was aware that in the course of his travels he had worn large holes in his shoes so his socks were visible and, since his threadbare socks could have finally disintegrated on the way to the interview, he might be displaying bare flesh. He explained that 'in any case, either socks or flesh would create an abominable impression, so that throughout the conversation I had to sit rigidly in an entirely unnatural position trying to remember, while chatting in an easy manner, to keep my feet flat on the carpet'. As if this was not enough he had to grip his wrists with his hands to conceal his frayed shirt cuffs.

The fellowship secured and his overdraft paid off by the first tranche of money from Queen's, my father compensated himself for the stress he had suffered during the interview by having four pairs of shoes and several silk shirts specially made for him. He chose Berlin over Vienna as the place to live because a friend offered him an introduction to *The Times* correspondent there. In the event the correspondent had departed two years earlier, so he telephoned his successor, Norman Ebbutt, at 8.30 a.m., hoping to give an impression of alertness. This might have been disastrous since Ebbutt, after a festive evening, had only just gone to bed. But being a good-natured man, he allowed my father to start writing articles for the paper and promoted his reputation with *The Times* back in London. Claud enjoyed the paper's high intellectual standards and touching self-importance, his account of which is usually quoted in any history of *The Times* of this era. He also impressed the powers that be at the newspaper by turning down their first three job offers, all involving a gradual rise through the ranks before reaching the rank of foreign correspondent. In fear that he might be about to torpedo any chance of working for the paper, he wrote to say he would like to be their correspondent so long as it could be in New York. Geoffrey Dawson, the editor of *The Times*, later an arch-exponent of appeasement and not a man with a reputation for warm-heartedness, in this case telegraphed immediately: 'HAVE NO FEAR FOR TOMORROW. RETURN AT ONCE. JOB WAITING.'

My father arrived in New York in the summer of 1929. He had spent a brief period in London at *The Times* on the way (where he contributed to Fleet Street folklore by winning a competition for the most boring headline with 'SMALL EARTHQUAKE IN CHILE. NOT MANY DEAD'). In Germany he had started reading the Marxist classics, predicting the downfall of capitalism. They dismissed the political assumptions on which he had been brought up as dangerous and self-serving delusions. He was impressed, but at the same time the German economy was prospering and across the Atlantic the US seemed to disprove everything written by Marx and Lenin. There was a rush of books in Berlin by liberals and socialists just returned from the US with titles like *Ford Answers Marx*. Workers and employers, instead of being locked in inevitable conflict, were getting rich together. The stock market surged higher every day and he found on his first day in New York that it was the only real topic of conversation: 'You could talk about prohibition, or Hemingway, or air conditioning, or music, or horses, but in the end you had to talk about the stock market, and that was where the conversation became serious.' Nor were you allowed to speak ill of its long-term prospects, whatever the short-term 'adjustments', in case by sympathetic magic you should jinx the great money-making machine. Through the hot summer months in Manhattan Claud wondered if Marx and his followers might not have got the future of the world very wrong. He did not have much time to think about it because his rapid promotion within *The Times* meant that he had to spend time learning how to write a basic news piece. His first copy was carefully written out in long hand because he did not know how to use a typewriter.

When the stock market crashed in October Claud found he had a ringside seat. He wrote a classic account of it in the first volume of his autobiography, *In Time of Trouble*. It was the event which led to the collapse of Germany and Austria and the rise of Hitler to power. It destroyed governments across the world. It took time for the enormity of the disaster to sink in. As my father was writing his dispatch on the first day of the crash, a fellow correspondent leaned forward and whispered to him: 'Remember, when we're writing this story the word "panic" is not to be used.' Claud recalled the story about the enthusiastic American and phlegmatic Englishman watching the great waterfall at Niagara. 'Isn't that amazing?' said the American. 'Look at that vast mass of water dashing over that enormous cliff!' The Englishman peered at the torrent for a few moments and then said: 'But what is to stop it?'

In the next few years it became clear that nothing was going to stop the political and economic reverberations of the crash around the world. Claud suddenly found himself, only months after learning to use a typewriter, summoned from New York to temporarily fill in for Sir Wilmott Lewis, *The Times* correspondent in Washington. My father regarded his understanding of journalism and American politics with deep respect, not least for one piece of journalistic advice. 'I think it well to remember,' Lewis told him, 'that when writing for the newspapers, we are writing for an elderly lady in Hastings who has two cats of which she is passionately fond. Unless our stuff can successfully compete for her interest with those cats, it is no good.'

It used to surprise and annoy my father in later years to be asked so frequently why he joined the Communist Party in 1933, soon after founding the *Week*. He had just seen the world he had grown up in collapse into ruin. The Nazis and Fascists were seizing power in central and southern Europe. Spain was soon engulfed in a savage civil war. The persecution of the Jews which was to lead to the death camps had already begun. In these circumstances he found it amazing not that he and so many others had become communists, but that there were people who could have watched these great disasters unmoved. He answered questions about why he joined and later left the party over many pages in his autobiography, but his account is complex and scattered in different parts of it. Readers seemed disappointed that there was not a pithier and shorter explanation as to why he had become a communist. There is in fact a crude but still adequate account of why he did so from a hostile source. Douglas Hyde, a British communist who later renounced the party, wrote a book called *I Believed*, denouncing his former comrades. But surprisingly he speaks of Claud in warm and approving terms and recounts several conversations with him:

He had only just arrived in the land where every bricklayer was said to have a car when the Wall Street crash came like a bolt from the blue.

'I had only to look out of my office window,' he told me, in characteristically colourful terms, 'to see stockbrokers and financiers jumping out of the windows on to the street below all day long.'

That was it. This was the collapse of Capitalism. After this should come the Revolution. Old man Marx was right after all. He threw up his job – and a promising career – to return to England and there to join the Communist Party.

He took a job on the the *Daily Worker* at not more than one twentieth of what he could earn on Fleet Street.[9]

In reality there were other highly practical reasons why my father became a communist and remained one until he departed for Ireland in 1947. It was not that he believed the communists had the answer to all humanity's problems. He thought rather that they were the only body which could effectively organise and fight for the poor and the powerless against the rich and powerful. In the 1930s he saw them as the one group which could combat the rising power of the Fascists and Nazis. When Claud relaunched his career as a professional humorist in the 1950s, his friends such as Malcolm Muggeridge wrote about him as having greater familiarity with P. G. Wodehouse than the works of Karl Marx. They played down his role in the party as an eccentric foible or a sign of his permanent opposition to the powers that be. *The Times*, his former employer, wrote sympathetically that it was 'symptomatic of that topsy-turvy period that so dyed-in-the-wool an individualist and debunker of important persons and orthodoxies should have thrown in his lot with comrades in a party that cared nothing for liberty or personal freedom and was devoid alike of pity and of humour'.[10] But his commitment to communism was more serious than they supposed. He believed that the communists alone had the capacity to contend for power on behalf of the dispossessed against their oppressors. His departure from the party was sparked as much by the communists' inability to fight effectively on behalf of the dispossessed whom they claimed to represent, as by the savage brutality of their rule in the Soviet Union and Eastern Europe. He was aware of the latter, having viewed during visits in the mid-1940s 'the chaos of Rumania, the comparative stagnation of Bulgaria, and above all, the arid desert of East Germany'.

Having decided to leave the party in 1947, he was also determined to do nothing which would bring joy to the heart of Senator McCarthy or appear as an endorsement of the opponents of communism. It never occurred to him, even at moments of greatest dearth, to write 'the familiar 50,000 words entitled "My fifteen years in a snakepit" which would certainly shake the coconut trees but be otherwise undesirable'. As it was, Claud's silent departure from the party, without any expressions of anger or disillusionment, would for several years mystify both his former comrades in the party and, it emerged many years later, the agents of MI5 who had assiduously followed his career for twenty years.

Eleven

My father left no private papers. They had been destroyed or lost over the years. There are the reminiscences of friends and enemies, but the only source of consecutive information about his life hitherto has been his own three-volume autobiography. The existence of a further well-informed and highly detailed source on his career emerged only a quarter of a century after his death in 1981. He had observed after he started the *Week* in 1933 that MI5, in charge of domestic security, was keeping a close eye on his activities. He rightly assumed that they opened his mail and listened to his telephone calls. Even so he would have been impressed and flattered by the twenty-six volumes of information about him released to the National Archives by MI5 in 2004. It begins with a trip Claud and Graham Greene took as students to the Rhineland, then occupied by British and French forces, in 1924. The purpose was to study local conditions and write about them on their return. They were regarded with suspicion by British intelligence because they failed to obtain visas and carried a letter of introduction from the German Foreign

Office in Berlin to the German authorities in Cologne. 'Both [men] appear to be authors,' wrote an intelligence officer dubiously.[1]

The MI5 files are packed with information, often absurdly detailed and compiled with immense labour by intelligence officers, policemen, informants and other intelligence agencies. All letters addressed to him were laboriously opened at the post office and a photostat made (though it soon became evident to MI5 officers that much of Claud's correspondence, and certainly anything that might be of interest to them, was sent to the houses of friends for collection). Phone calls at his office and home were intercepted and conversations transcribed. Plain-clothes men waited for him when he left home in the morning and followed him until his return in the evening. The original purpose of this prolonged pursuit was to find out his contacts and the sources for stories appearing in the *Week*. The close surveillance continued, perhaps through bureaucratic momentum, long after it was clear that it was producing nothing of value. If officers from MI5 were truly interested in finding his sources then they were uniformly unsuccessful. Had they done so there was not much they could have done about them because so many of his stories came from other journalists unable to publish them in their own newspapers.

Useless though this plodding accumulation of facts may have been for any practical purpose, they give a unique and detailed portrait of Claud's life which would have been impossible to emulate even if he and his friends had been meticulous diarists. No piece of trivia is too irrelevant to record. Here, for instance, is the account of the Special Branch man, who refers to himself as 'the Watcher', following my father on 30 March 1940 when he took my mother, then Mrs Patricia Byron, on a visit to Tring in Hertfordshire, where he had partly been brought up, and nearby Berkhamsted where he went to school. The policeman evidently had no idea of the reason for the trip.

On Saturday, 30th March, Cockburn left home at noon, and after visiting the 'Adam & Eve' P.H. walked to St James's Park Station where he telephoned and examined a map of the Green Line Coach Service. At 12.20 p.m. he entered the 'Feathers' P.H. remaining till 12.55 p.m. He then returned home. At 2.15 p.m. he left with the young woman believed to be Mrs Patricia Byron with whom he had been seen before at 84, Buckingham Gate. They went to the Victoria Coaching Station, and then to the Green Line Coach Station, Eccleston Bridge, and they travelled by the 2.34 p.m. coach and alighted just before reaching Tring. They then climbed a hill and entered a wood close to Lord Rothschild's Estate. At this point our Watcher was forced to drop out owing to the risk of detection, but at 6.00 p.m. the couple were picked up having tea in the 'Rose & Crown Inn', Tring. At 6.30 p.m. they left and travelled by bus to Berkhamsted, arriving at 6.50 p.m. They walked around town, and along the canal tow path, and eventually reached the 'King's Arms' P.H. where they entered at 7.10 p.m. At 8.15 p.m. they left and boarded an 8.20 p.m. Green Line Coach, but alighted at Watford, where they entered another P.H. at 8.50 p.m. where they remained till 9.10 p.m. then walked to Watford Town Station, and travelled by the 9.25

p.m. train for St James's Park Station, changing at Charing Cross, and then walked to 84, Buckingham Gate where they entered at 10.40 p.m.

It may be stated that Cockburn is a heavy drinker of whisky.

Description of his woman companion (believed Byron):– age 26; height 5'2"; slim build; dark rather long hair; sharp features; cultured voice; dressed in blue costume and brown coat; black low heeled shoes; no hat.

Observation continuing as circumstances permit.[2]

Comment on the staggering amount my father could drink – my mother stuck to gin and tonic and was a far more moderate consumer – is a recurring feature in these MI5 reports. On occasion they would record hopefully that he had become a full-time alcoholic. Sometimes there is a tone of strong disapproval. As late as February 1951, when he was visiting London from Ireland, an official memo noted: 'It was learnt that he was an extremely unpopular guest at the Park Lane Hotel where in particular his behaviour in the Bar caused umbrage both to the management and other customers.'[3] He always drank heavily, but he had a naturally strong constitution. When he was medically examined for military service in 1943 he was found to be in perfect health. Aside from the drinking, he smoked several packs of cigarettes a day yet he survived TB in both lungs, cancer of the throat and numerous other ailments to die at the age of seventy-seven.

The replacement of the letter by the telephone as the main means of communication is said to have made it more difficult to write a good biography in the twentieth century than in the nineteenth century. Too many critical exchanges take place on the telephone and are unrecorded. (In the twenty-first century email means that once again important communications may be preserved for historians.) In my father's case, however, his phone calls were faithfully transcribed at the post office. These intercepts at least provided MI5 with a list of his contacts, though they produced little other valuable information. Going by the reports of the Special Branch officers following him, Claud made sensitive calls from public phone boxes or obtained information in face-to-face meetings usually taking place in pubs. Some of the phone intercepts, transcribed regardless of who was on the phone or what they were talking about, carry a touching sense of intimacy. In June 1948, for instance, Claud was talking to Patricia when 'Claud's small son [my brother Alexander aged seven] then came to the 'phone and particularly requested his father to get home early as he wanted him to read a new book nurse had bought him about Christopher Robin. Claud told him that he thought he couldn't read it that evening as he had some friends coming but promised to read the following day.'[4]

Angry internal memos and minutes preserved by MI5 underline the invulnerability and anonymity previously enjoyed by civil servants and the outrage they felt at seeing their names in print. In the summer of 1935 Claud wrote an attack on a consular official called Preston. 'To attack a civil servant by name is a cad's trick,' wrote an official called C. C. Farrer, who noted in an aggrieved tone that 'not so long ago he published a War Office circular which was marked, and was, Secret'. Other officials, mostly from the Foreign Office, mulled over various methods by which they might 'make it very hot for the paper'. But, though tempted, they also reflected that any action on their part would only give publicity to the *Week*. One official noted that when a similar case involving the newsletter had arisen previously, 'we considered taking legal action but were advised that the rag had no assets and would gain by the publicity'.[5] Civil servants on occasion showed strenuous enthusiasm for action to be taken against the *Week*, so long as it was taken by somebody else. At one moment Sir Robert Vansittart, the permanent secretary at the Foreign Office, is reported to have been 'extremely angry' and wanted the Director of Public Prosecutions to prosecute. The DPP said 'this was out of the question, and he definitely turned down the possibility of doing anything in the nature of warning Claud Cockburn'. The internal debate is concluded by a note from Captain Liddell of MI5, wryly quoting Virgil on the unhappiness in the Foreign Office and their frustration at their inability to do anything about it: 'As for the F.O.: "Sedet aeturnumque sedebit infelix Dido."' (Sits and will forever sit unhappy Dido).[6] In other words, the moaning from the Foreign Office, while persistent, was going to get its members precisely nowhere.

The great mass of information accumulated by MI5 suffers from the shortcoming typical of so many official files. There is too much detail. Interesting though this is to a historian, an official reading it would have difficulty distinguishing between pieces of gossip and reliable facts. There is a natural tendency for a rumour or an exaggeration to acquire credibility when it gets into an official file and is read at the same time as more authentic information. Asked to write a memo on, in this case, my father, officials understandably tended to reduce their workload to the minimum by borrowing as much as they could from previous memos. For instance, in 1939 a document by a private inquiry agent on my father was sent on to MI5 from Naval Intelligence, claiming to have information about a sinister 'Cockburn machine', marked as coming from 'a certain Mr Prior who was a friend of Pay Cap Jerram, Admiral Chatfield's secretary'. It is a strange mixture of well-known information and spy-fiction fantasy. It claims Cockburn is 'one of the most important men working for the Comintern in Western Europe. He is responsible for all political information and the "Cockburn Machine" as it is referred to controls military, naval and industrial espionage and would be responsible for sabotage in the event of war or revolution.'[7] Doubts about Mr Prior's grasp on current political events are increased when he reveals that he considers *Time* magazine in New York as secretly answering to the Communist International. He says darkly at the end of his letter that a 'conservative Member for Aberdeen is in the Cockburn organisation'. Officials were not inclined to take this too seriously. 'Is this information of alleged enquiry agents of any use to you or any other Govt. Dept?' one asks lazily. 'If not, I think I had better tell him so tactfully.' As the years passed, however, other officials called to write a quick memo about Claud began cheerfully to incorporate the dubious information in this submission by Mr Prior into their memoranda. (Journalists behave in exactly the same way. Called on to write a piece for immediate publication, they crib without attribution stories of whose veracity they have no direct knowledge from their own or other newspapers. This is why it is so difficult to eliminate errors once they have crept into the journalistic food chain, particularly as invented stories are likely to be juicier than the more prosaic truth.)

The analysis by MI5 and Foreign Office officials was generally shallow, but their hunger for information was unending. This ensured the survival of interesting titbits of information. There is an intercepted telegram from Claud in 1937 reading 'MINE IMPEDES PROGRESS', after the ship he was sailing on struck a mine off the Spanish coast.[8] Four years later in the summer of 1941 my mother, heavily pregnant, was staying in Ross-shire in Scotland. She wrote to Claud, according to a letter copied by MI5, that 'she feels depressed and is expecting her baby in two months' time. Thanks him for speaking to her over the phone, and begs him to do so again, as often as he can.'

Curious episodes in my father's memoir are sometimes confirmed. In the early days of the *Week* he complained that he was troubled by enthusiastic people proffering help he did not need. A man from Vancouver said he could get lots of advertising and was generally instructive on the business of launching a newsletter. Claud recalled: 'He stayed with us, in fact, throughout the launching of the paper and for three weeks after it had begun to come out, but then he went out of his mind just outside the Army and Navy stores where he knelt on the pavement one morning, addressing me as his Brother in the Sun.' An MI5 memo on 'Claud Cockburn and "The Week"', composed soon after the newsletter was launched in the spring of 1933, noted that 'T. B. F. Sheard, shown as manager, is no longer employed. He had a particularly sharp bout of what is known as "financial irresponsibility", in the course of which he removed the funds.'[9] This was Benvenuto Sheard, the Oxford friend who had loaned Claud the forty pounds to start the *Week*. MI5 knew about what happened because they had intercepted and copied a begging letter from Claud to Nancy Cunard asking her to make up the shortfall in funds. The letter reads: 'Dear Nancy, the following has happened. Sheard (Manager of the *Week*) has had a complete breakdown, break up, preceded as I now find by a short but peculiarly sharp burst of what is called "financial irresponsibility". I.e. he has got away with the entire funds, accumulated during the first four issues.'[10] Another official minute mentions that Sheard after 'a brainstorm' had even written to King George V, whom he asked 'to interest his influential friends' on behalf of the paper.

The interest of MI5 in my father essentially starts with the foundation of the *Week*. As mentioned above, the only documents of an earlier date in his file relate to his visit to Germany in 1924 with Graham Greene when they were both students. But within three months of the *Week* being published in 1933 a Michael Wright from the Foreign Office rang up MI5, the domestic security service founded by Colonel Sir Vernon Kell in 1909 and run by him until 1940. An officer recorded: 'Mr Wright said that a great deal of what was in the paper was all right, but that Cockburn appeared to be getting information from someone in Government Departments.'[11] MI5 soon had a fairly accurate picture of my father's career. It said that before departing *The Times*, he had told his chief in

213

New York 'that he had a mission in life, but did not explain what he meant'. Civil servants in the intelligence service sound perplexed on how seriously they should take the *Week,* saying 'it is a curious farrago of would-be clever cynical inside information, mainly on foreign affairs. Sometimes COCKBURN appears to be singularly well-informed on matters of a confidential Government nature, but so far it has not been possible to establish exactly how far this may be due to some leakage, or to intelligent anticipation.'

The official tone is often snooty. At one point a memo remarks: 'He is also known to have associations with many far from desirable elements in the lower walks of journalistic life.' This is combined with high respect for his abilities: 'I think it is only reasonable to state that COCKBURN is a man whose intelligence and capability, combined with his Left Wing tendencies and an unscrupulous nature, make him a formidable factor with which to reckon.'[12] A three-page résumé of his career written in 1934 by an inspector in the Special Branch, though it contains some mistakes, came to broadly the same conclusion. The inspector writes: 'I am informed that so much is thought of the ability of F. Claud COCKBURN that he could return to the staff of The Times any day he wished, if he would keep his work to the desired policy of this newspaper. By his former colleagues on the "Times" he is regarded more as a clever fool than a dangerous knave.' The inspector, who had evidently spent some time in Fleet Street, wrote: 'He is a daring commentator, and has also been described to me as a professional mischief maker, who delights in making mischief.'[13] The Special Branch believed that Claud was associating more and more with communists.

Telephone calls to and from the tiny one-room office at 34 Victoria Street were intercepted and a list of contacts compiled. Jean Ross was a frequent caller. A charming, cultured woman, she lived with my father between 1933 and 1939 and was the mother of my half-sister Sarah. An MI5 official wrote of her: 'Cockburn's ablest assistant in his work on "The Week" is Jean Ross. She was with Cockburn in Madrid during the early stages of the Spanish Civil War and has subsequently been largely responsible for the publication of "The Week".'[14] Jean gained notoriety – she felt unfairly – because of a chance encounter when she had been working as an actress in Berlin in 1931. She had briefly shared a small flat with Christopher Isherwood and to her surprise he later claimed her as the model for Sally Bowles in *Goodbye to Berlin*. The stage version was called *I Am a Camera* and it was made into the award-winning film *Cabaret* in which Liza Minnelli portrays Sally Bowles as an empty-headed vamp. Jean did not in any way identify with Sally Bowles and suspected that Isherwood had really modelled the character on one of his boyfriends, but dared not admit that he was homosexual. My sister Sarah, a barrister and later a writer of detective stories, believed that Isherwood, supposedly avant-garde, was in practice highly conventional. Her point was that 'convention requires that a woman must be either virtuous (in the sexual sense) or a tart. So Sally, who is not virtuous, must be a tart.'

To find out what was happening at the *Week*, two MI5 agents posing as would-be contributors visited the office at different times. It must have been a comic scene. Neither agent can have been very convincing. They had to pretend, still puffing after the climb up the endless stairs at

34 Victoria Street, that they had dropped by almost on a whim to see the editor. The first informer did not even succeed in this and saw only the two secretaries. They told him Claud was not in and only dropped by occasionally. The agent was a little aggrieved by these irregular office hours. He reported tetchily to his controller that 'it seems remarkable that the editor of this paper should only visit his editorial offices for half an hour a day'.[15]

The agents' reports exude a sleazy zeal to please their masters by offering up titbits of useless information such as half-overheard telephone conversations. A second informant did get to see Claud on 2 November 1933. He said: 'He swallowed my story and asked for an article, which I shall accordingly prepare today. He is either very crafty or very gullible, for he invited me to have a boozing evening with him tomorrow, which I cannot unfortunately afford in present circumstances to do, and therefore invented an appointment.'[16] Five days later the first part-time agent had tea with my father: 'He told me he thought war very imminent, so much so that "if I polish my S.B. [Sam Browne] belt for Armistice Day I shan't need to polish it again for mobilisation". He thinks the Far East the likeliest spot.' The agent claimed that Claud was on occasion naive and ill-informed, but the fact that he twice asked MI5's man 'who had put me on to him' suggests that he was suspicious of this chance visitor. His prediction of imminent conflict is in keeping with a mischievous habit he had of telling people who were trying to pump him or whom he simply found boring that war or revolution were likely within days. In November 1945, during a visit to Bulgaria, a British diplomat he spoke to wrote home in agitation that Claud and Patricia 'are dangerous. She is of the proselytising type and earnest. He is a good listener.' Claud had alarmed the diplomat by telling him about the extent of infiltration of the Labour Party.[17] On another occasion an outraged woman wrote to some contact at MI5 saying that she had sat next to Claud at dinner and he had predicted imminent revolution beginning in the Brigade of Guards.

Not all security inquiries were so footling. In 1935 Colonel Valentine Vivian, the head of counter-espionage at MI6, wrote to Captain Liddell at MI5 saying he had sent MI6's man in Berlin to talk to Norman Ebbutt, the correspondent of *The Times*. It was Ebbutt who had launched my father's career and he was happy to discuss what had happened. He said 'he discovered Cockburn in 1926, and was so impressed by his brilliant intelligence that he appointed him to his staff. He soon became aware of the political sympathies of COCKBURN, who was a frequent visitor to communist meetings and had friends in that party, but retained his services on the understanding that he would keep his views out of the paper. He was hoping that Cockburn would change with time.' Ebbutt arranged for him to be transferred to London. Soon afterwards in the US he said he could no longer conceal his real views and asked to resign. The MI6 agent in Berlin reported the conversation:

Some of the 'Times' leading men, who were then in Washington – I think they were Sir W. Lewis, Dawson and Deakin – appealed to him not to be silly and reiterated Ebbutt's grounds of appeal, viz: that he should not destroy a brilliant career by openly adopting communist tenets. He replied that he could not help himself: he was a convinced communist; he felt he had to sacrifice everything for his convictions.

Ebbutt has the highest opinion of COCKBURN's honesty and admires him for feeding on the crust of an idealist when he could obtain a fat appointment by being untrue to himself ... Ebbutt says 'The Week' has a large circulation among businessmen in the City. He gets his copy regularly. He very much regrets that COCKBURN has now completely fallen to the mad idea that all Imperialists dream of nothing but the destruction of Russia.[18]

By the time they talked to Ebbut both MI5 and MI6 already knew Claud had become a communist. His contact with the communists was at first through the National Council for Civil Liberties, support for which led to him being arrested for the only time in his life. The government banned meetings outside labour exchanges. The NCCL challenged the ruling by breaking the ban. On 1 August 1934 Claud and a man called Robert McLennan tried to speak near Battersea Park. A police inspector stopped them. According to the lengthy Special Branch notes of the police court hearings a few days later, 'Cockburn then pushed in between McLennan and the inspector and said: "I am from the Council of Civil Liberties. I demand to know why we can't hold a meeting."' A crowd of two hundred gathered and shouted: 'This is Fascism.' On refusing to move away, Claud and McLennan were arrested and spent the night in jail.'[19] As he moved towards the communists he wrote his first story for the *Daily Worker* on the Gresford mining disaster in North Wales in September 1934. When the war in Spain broke out he covered it for the *Daily Worker* under the name of Frank Pitcairn.

Generally Claud was philosophical about MI5 and Special Branch surveillance. Yet another MI5 agent, referred to as 'M7', who visited the *Week* had a long conversation with his secretary. 'She referred to the difficulties of evading the government's spy system and said that of course their letters are all opened,' reported the informant. 'This was a nuisance rather than a danger, for it meant that every Monday morning COCKBURN had to make a tour of friends' houses picking up letters which they dared not have sent to the office.'[20] Only occasionally is there a snap of irritation on Claud's part. In the autumn of 1935 he complained in the *Week* about intrusive measures taken to add to his dossier: 'For a while not a man, woman or child who visited the editor's flat at any hour of the day or night escaped the distinction of being entered in the dossier and "further investigated".' A politically innocent woman friend came under surveillance and the surveillance team compiled 'a really fine list of elderly ladies and gentlemen, actually her uncles and aunts but henceforth suspect of heaven knows what international conspiracy'.[21]

Once Claud became publicly identified with the communists, MI5 officials seem relieved that they were no longer dealing with an unknown political quantity. References to him are generally respectful. In the spring of 1937 Colonel Sir Vernon Kell wrote a note on Claud to a diplomat at the American Embassy in London, saying:

'Cockburn is a man whose intelligence and wide variety of contacts make him a formidable factor on the side of Communism.'[22] He complained that the *Week* was full of gross inaccuracies and was written from a left-wing point of view, but admitted that, on occasion, 'he is quite well informed and by intelligent anticipation gets quite close to the truth'. At the end of the previous year a memo sent to MI5 noted that the circulation of the newsletter had risen sharply because of an article 'dealing with the relationship between His Majesty the King and Mrs E. Simpson'.[23]

Interest in Claud intensified again in the first year of the war as the *Week* followed the party line in opposing the war. There was an internal debate among officials about suppressing it entirely. Some argued that instead the editor should be tried for sedition by a judge and jury: 'Otherwise its traitorous supporters can run about the country saying (a) that the Government is a foul tyranny and (b) that they have got the government rattled.'[24] Given that these discussions were going on when London was being bombed nightly by the German air force, this unwillingness to use emergency powers unless compelled to do so shows impressive restraint.

In January 1941 the *Week* was suppressed. The Special Branch reported with satisfaction of Claud that 'at present he is penniless and heavily in debt'. A few months later they added that he had become 'a somewhat disgruntled man' and lacked an outlet for his journalistic capabilities. They wondered if they should give him a pass to visit Patricia, pregnant with my brother Alexander, in Ross-shire which was a closed military area. This involved a prolonged search of Somerset

House to see if the two were in fact married.[25] This was a question to which much official time was devoted. In June the Special Branch wrote uncertainly that 'it appears likely that she married him on 13 February 1941. It may be of interest that she describes her father as Major John Bernard Arbuthnot.'[26]

It was only when my mother died in 1989 that it was discovered that for some reason my parents had never married during the war or, for that matter, for many years afterwards. Among Patricia's papers was a wedding certificate showing that they had got married on 20 March 1978 in Westminster. They were staying with me in my flat at 90 Westbourne Terrace near Paddington at the time, while Claud was having successful radiation treatment for throat cancer. He died three years later. Under a heading on the form marked 'condition', the registrar in Westminster has written: 'Previously went through a form of marriage at Sofia, Bulgaria on the 2nd March 1946.' I do not know why they did not get married earlier but it may have been due to some delay in my mother's divorce from Arthur Byron. She had in the early days of the war gone to some trouble to conceal the fact that she and Claud were not married by changing her name by deed poll to 'Patricia Cockburn'.

Two years later officials debated at length whether Claud should be called up for military service. In a lengthy memo one official concluded that 'Cockburn is an exceedingly clever man, who takes good care to keep within the law and, while his literary output is contentious and carping, it cannot be considered a subversive activity'. On the other hand, if he was enlisted in the armed services and refrained from subversive actions 'he would almost inevitably be selected for commissioned rank, and, apart from possible subversive activities, he would have access to much secret information which, in view of his former activities as a Comintern agent, would be highly undesirable'.[27]

My father's delicate steps out of the Communist Party and his move to Ireland confused both MI5 and the party leaders for a surprisingly long time. He was in fact trying to work for different publications under different names. My mother complained in a phone call not that her calls were intercepted but that MI5 gossiped about the contents of the calls, thus exposing what noms de plume Claud was using. In 1949 the Communist leaders worried that he was about to follow Douglas Hyde, the veteran party member, and convert to Roman Catholicism. The *Daily Express* called up Harry Pollitt, the general secretary of the British Communist Party, to enquire whether Claud was still a party member. An agitated Pollitt soon afterwards had a comic conversation with another party leader named Johnnie Campbell. The phone intercept reads:

Harry says his fear is the Catholic business.

Johnnie says he has not much to fear on that. 'She' (?) is a member of the Protestant Ascendancy [my mother]. The old Protestant . . . Ireland families. For them to go Catholic is almost as bad as a South American Senator marrying a negress.

Harry says oh! He says they will keep their fingers crossed. Johnnie says he could get Derek (Kartun) over here to spy out the land if he thought it worthwhile.

Harry thinks it is worthwhile. It is worth the money to be on guard.

Johnnie says O.K.[28]

A man who had been sent to Youghal by the William Hickey column in the *Daily Express* ran my father to earth at Brook Lodge, but he refused to say if he had left the party. 'I have absolutely no statement to make. I consider the question impertinent.' The *Express* journalist watched Claud bicycling into Youghal and back: 'Now and then he drops into the Royal Bar for an Irish whiskey. Then he pedals home, head down against wind, against rain. And against the party line . . . ?'[29] Slower on the uptake, the Special Branch reported a few months later that 'Cockburn has profound disagreements with the Communist Party. Curiously enough, these are alleged to be principally over the question of Lysenko [the fraudulent biologist befriended by Stalin].'[30] A first cousin of Claud's called George Cruikshank even wrote from Singapore, saying: 'Family rumour has it that he has joined or is about to join the Catholic Church. If this is true, I should think it most unlikely that is a faked conversion. He was very seriously ill about three years ago, when he was also shaken by his mother's death.'[31] MI5 turned to Douglas Hyde, a genuine defector, who had run into Claud, who completely ignored him, in Ireland. Hyde had sensibly made enquiries with the local parish priest in Youghal, 'who informed him that Cockburn showed no signs of conversion to Roman Catholicism. Hyde's own view is that Cockburn may have severed his connections with the Party without necessarily ceasing to be a Communist.'[32]

During all this time the machinery of surveillance rolled on. Every time Claud travelled between Ireland and Britain the Special Branch conducted a 'discreet search' of his luggage and reported to MI5. The last volume of the enormous file on my father ends in 1953. The overall impression of twenty years of the industrious chronicling of his activities by MI5 is that a clear picture of my father's character and activities are submerged in a vast accumulation of details. There is a failure to distinguish between the important and the trivial, and between the reliable and the unreliable. It is as if intelligence officials found reassurance in the sheer bulk of the information they had acquired. In their defence it could be said that they did not put this information to any very sinister use such as arresting or interning him, which they could easily have done in the early years of the war.

What did the communists think of my father, about whose abilities MI5 wrote such laudatory reviews? Since the fall of the Soviet Union it is possible to look at the Comintern files stored in the Russian State Archive of Social and Political History in Bolshaya Dmitrovka Street in Moscow. The documents on Claud are sparse compared to the great archive compiled by British intelligence. But they do contain one surprising disclosure which my father would have found amusing and ironical. At almost the same moment that Colonel Sir Vernon Kell was telling the Americans that Claud 'was a formidable factor on the side of Communism', the Comintern chiefs in the Soviet Union were trying to sack him. His crimes were deviations from the party line and the belief in Moscow that he had cut a crucial part of an interview given by Stalin. 'We know him from the negative point of view,' wrote a Comintern official in Moscow called Bilov in a secret memo on Claud written on 25 May 1937.[33] These were ominous words at a moment when the great purges were gathering steam across the Soviet Union and far smaller or non-existent errors had fatal results for their supposed perpetrators. Bilov goes on to explain that 'in the middle of 1936 we suggested to the English Communist Party to sack Cockburn from the senior editorial management as one of the people responsible for the systematic appearance of different types of "mistakes" of a purely provocative character on the pages of the *Daily Worker*'.

From the beginning the party was a little bewildered by its new recruit, though they swiftly recognised his effectiveness. In 1936–7 party officials in London working for the Comintern, supposedly uniting all Communist Parties, wrote a series of reports about him to the leadership in Moscow. They contained admiring comments. One said: 'He is held to be one of Fleet Street's cleverest journalists.'[34] Another noted his ability to reveal changes in the Cabinet before they were announced: 'He is in touch with bankers and other elements who are in close touch with what goes on in the bourgeois camp and Government circles.'[35] But the reports have the edgy tone of inquisitors looking for heretics in the ranks. One report in 1936 refers to Jean Ross, saying Harry Pollitt 'distrusts this woman but has no facts to connect her with the enemy'.[36]

There were more specific criticisms. One report reads:

The mistakes recently made in the *Daily Worker* on

the question of the Chinese students' agitation and the omission of a vital part of Comrade Stalin's interview with Ron Howard are to be attributed in the first place to Cockburn. More recently in one of his early dispatches from Spain, where he is working as *Daily Worker* correspondent, the bad mistake was made of depicting the Communists and the socialist workers' organisations as seizing on the present events to install a regime of socialism.[37]

Of these deviations the only one that seemed to matter was the sub-editing of Stalin's words; another Soviet official was still complaining about it ten years later.

By 1953 MI5 seems to have accepted that Claud was no longer connected with the party. His old friend Otto Katz, the Mayor of Prague, had been executed after confessing that he had been recruited to British intelligence by a certain Colonel Cockburn. (More than twenty years earlier MI5 had noticed that Katz had been appointed the Paris correspondent of a British newspaper through Claud's influence.)[38] The Hungarian uprising and the Suez crisis were establishing a new pattern of Cold War politics, and he was openly working under his own name at *Punch*. The lumbering machinery of surveillance which had observed Claud for so long finally ground to a halt.

Twelve

I did not think all that much about the polio epidemic in Cork in 1956 until over forty years later in Iraq. I was in Baghdad to write about the latest American bombardment ordered by President Bill Clinton at the end of 1998. The city was blacked out and the anti-aircraft fire twinkled like fireflies in the night sky. Every few minutes an American missile would explode, sending up a spout of fire. As I sat by the open window in my room in the Al-Rashid hotel I could feel warm gusts of air from the blasts brush against my cheek. I could clearly hear the excited chatter of a television correspondent reporting live from a room next to me. His exaggerated description of the proximity of the explosions to the hotel made them feel almost unreal to me and I felt less threatened.

The next day we visited hospitals to talk to the wounded from the overnight attacks. I was walking down a ward, the beds filled with injured children, wondering how their lives would be affected by the events of the night, when I began to remember St Finbarr's and Gurranebraher hospitals in Cork. It suddenly seemed strange to me that I should spend so many years as a journalist covering other people's crises, yet I knew so little about the disaster which had had such an impact on my own life. I did not at that stage even know the exact year in which the epidemic had taken place.

I do not mean that I had not thought about the effect of having polio in all the years between 1956 and 1998. In one sense I thought about it all the time. It was part of my identity. I cannot run, I do not drive and I have a severe limp. But I did not think very much about how and why I had got polio. It was an event which existed outside time in my mind. No doubt there was an element of suppression in this. I did not want to recall unhappy memories. I was influenced by Patricia, Claud and Kitty Lee, all of whom, more than most people, consciously avoided dwelling on the past on the sensible grounds that there was nothing one could do to change it.

There was another reason why I did not have a clear picture of the epidemic. My knowledge of it consisted of the vivid but disjointed memories of a six-year-old child. I could remember Dr Gowen and the cold feel of his stethoscope on my chest on the day he came to Brook Lodge to diagnose me. I recalled my feeling of bewilderment and misery as I was lifted into the back of a cream-coloured ambulance parked on the drive by a dark green yew tree outside the front door of Brook Lodge. Later in St Finbarr's there was the smell of antiseptic and warm rubber. I had never forgotten my feeling of terror in Gurranebraher when I thought the nurses would force me to eat my own shit.

The American air attacks on Iraq in 1998, known collectively as 'Desert Fox', were soon over. It was one of the less significant episodes in the long-drawn-out Iraq crisis, which I wrote about for a quarter of a century. (The journalists and Iraqi officials in Baghdad cynically believed the bombardment had taken place so President Clinton could divert attention away from his impending impeachment by Congress over his affair with Monica Lewinsky.) But, as I drove out of Baghdad to return to Jordan and then by air to Ireland for Christmas, the thought remained with me that I should try to find out as much as I could about the epidemic and what had happened to me. My parents did not speak about polio very much. By the time I became interested in it they were both dead, my father, after surviving many illnesses, in 1981, and my mother in 1989. Kitty Lee did describe to me what had happened before she died in 2001. Unfortunately, a few years earlier she had thrown away letters about me that my mother had sent her when I was in hospital in London. 'I didn't see the point in keeping them,' she said. 'It was all in the past.' My father wrote a moving chapter about the epidemic in the third volume of his autobiography, *View from the West*. My mother has a brief and less revealing account in her memoir *Figure of Eight*.

I was not sure at first about the accuracy of my father's recollections. His book had been written in peculiarly strenuous circumstances. Soon after I had returned to Brook Lodge from hospital he was diagnosed as suffering from TB in both lungs. He went to a sanatorium in Cork where he wrote part of *View from the West* lying in an isolation cubicle. But his memory of what had happened to us turned out to be very clear. A look at the files of local newspapers showed that he had been quite right in

229

believing that the local press had suppressed news about polio from about ten weeks into the epidemic. By the time I caught it at the end of September nothing about the disease was being printed. As I sat in Cork library looking at microfilm of copies of old newspapers from 1956, I found it peculiarly evocative of the fear felt by the political and business establishment in Cork at the time that they had censored news about the epidemic at the moment I was lying in the back of an ambulance speeding towards St Finbarr's.

Almost nothing was written about the epidemic in the years that followed. Encyclopedias of Irish history find room to mention obscure skirmishes in the Elizabethan wars or describe the career of some harmless nineteenth-century Member of Parliament. But they say nothing about what happened in Cork in 1956 despite the fact that it paralysed the second-largest city in the country for a year. Almost the only written account is a succinct but unpublished account of the epidemic in a chapter in an excellent MA thesis by Fiona Wallace on voluntary provision for the disabled in Cork.[1] Perhaps one reason why the epidemic has been ignored is because it did not fit neatly into the usual categories of political, economic or social history. I wrote an essay on how I caught polio and about the epidemic of 1956 for the *Independent* magazine in the summer of 1999. I always intended to write more about it but in the autumn of that year I moved from Jerusalem to Moscow as correspondent covering the former Soviet Union. The second Chechen war was beginning and I was mostly engaged in writing about that bloody conflict. After the suicide plane attacks in New York on 11 September 2001 I went straight to Afghanistan and, after the fall of the Taliban, I began to write about Iraq which I had been visiting for years. I spent the months before and during the US-led invasion in Iraqi Kurdistan and it was only in the late summer of 2003 that I was able to start once again contacting doctors, nurses and patients involved in the Cork epidemic.

I was interested in why the polio epidemic in Cork had disappeared so entirely from written history. Dr Kathleen O'Callaghan, the cool-headed doctor at St Finbarr's, told me she believed the reason for the lack of published information was simple terror: 'People were that frightened at the time that they tried to forget it. I would see people cross the road rather than walk past the walls of the fever hospital.'[2] My father recalled that some bedridden people in Cork had nearly starved to death because it was thought they had polio and nobody would go near their houses to deliver milk, meat or vegetables. The police had to be called in to make the deliveries.

There was no shortage of other reminders of the epidemic in the shape of survivors in wheelchairs or callipers. It was this, perhaps, which made people so afraid of the disease and unwilling to talk about it. Its effects were very visible. Polio did not kill many people but it left them maimed. In 1994/95 there were between 7,500 and 10,000 survivors of the illness still alive in Ireland.[3] Tuberculosis, which my father contracted, had been prevalent in Ireland and was a far worse killer than polio. But my father, when he was released from his sanatorium, did not look any different from other people though his health never really recovered. He was not, like so many polio survivors, a walking advertisement for the effects of the disease.

231

I could understand why nobody in Cork wanted to hear about the epidemic because for a long time I did not want to hear about it myself. It is a natural enough human reaction to deal with disasters by trying to forget them. Even those crippled by polio often did not want to think about it or react to it very much. Calamity teaches endurance and a central part of endurance is a muting of the emotions and a filtering out of unhappy memories. Many years later in Belfast in 1974 at the height of the bombings and sectarian killings I remember expressing shock to Paddy Devlin, a friend who was an MP for the Social Democratic and Labour Party, about some murderous attack which had left many people dead and injured. He replied impatiently:

You don't really feel that. We all say in Belfast how shocked we are by some atrocity but it is not really true. Nobody who lives here with so many people being shot or blown apart every day can have an emotional reaction to every death. The truth is we don't really feel anything unless something happens to a member of our family or the half-dozen people we are closest to.

Even when recalling catastrophes long past there is a subconscious desire to keep a certain distance from them. For instance, people in the Blackwater valley would sometimes lament the impact of the Great Famine of the 1840s on the area, but then add that their own village was little affected though local records showed that the dead were so numerous that they had to be buried in pits.

Fear may have stopped people writing about the epi-

demic in the years immediately after 1956 but as the immediate sense of threat receded they might have become more
open about what had happened. By then, however, polio
had become part of ancient history because mass vaccination with the Salk vaccine had almost entirely eradicated it.

Reticence about the epidemic in the late 1950s had
another source which is peculiarly Irish, or at least different from the reaction in the US or the rest of Western
Europe. There was acute embarrassment that polio was
a sign of underdevelopment, one more indication that the
national independence of Ireland had failed to create a
modern nation. Irish self-confidence at the time was not
robust. As the rest of Western Europe recovered from the
war, Ireland was falling further behind and every year
more people emigrated to the US or Britain.

The most detailed articles on polio in the *Cork
Examiner* sought to disprove that people from the city
were spreading it elsewhere. Otherwise the victims are
never named. Dr Saunders, the able Medical Officer of
Health, had written a testy letter published in the press
to prove that Raymond Smith, the young seaman with
polio who had passed through Cork on his way to
Liverpool, must have contracted the disease earlier. Half
a century later doctors commonly publicise and even exaggerate the severity of an epidemic, such as CJD or SARS,
to ensure maximum publicity, early diagnosis and state
funding. In Cork in 1956 the doctors did not, at least at
first, want to suppress all news, but they did want to control it and play down the severity of the epidemic.

The paucity of written sources on the epidemic soon
became evident. All my own medical records had been

233

destroyed along with those of other patients. The only official record was an entry in the register in St Finbarr's showing the dates that I had entered and left the hospital. The destruction of records largely took place in the 1960s and 1970s and has no more sinister explanation than the need for storage space. This was before knowledge became widespread of post-polio syndrome, the weakening of muscles that afflicts survivors later in life because of hidden damage done by the virus so many years before. Such destruction of documents would be unlikely to take place today if only because litigation over past mistreatment in state institutions has become common.

When I first started investigating the epidemic I realised that if I was to find out about polio in Cork in 1956 I would have to do so as fast as possible. It had happened forty-three years earlier and fewer and fewer of the nurses and doctors who fought the epidemic were still alive. Survivors were far more numerous because almost all were very young when they caught it. But because they were so young they knew, like myself, very little about the general course of the disease or its effects on the city. It soon became apparent, however, that almost everybody in Cork alive at the time had been affected by the epidemic either because one of their relatives had got it or because they had been evacuated as children to other parts of Ireland. Donal O'Donovan, a civil servant working for the County Medical Officer of Health, compiled a weekly register of people with notifiable infections, including polio. He noticed a strange aspect of the disease: 'The thing I remember most about the epidemic in Cork is that about 95 per cent of the cases occurred in the more well-to-do suburbs like Douglas and Bishopstown.'[4] He realised – as few did in Cork at the time – that the poorer parts of the city were being spared.

It took me a long time to get better – or as well as I was ever going to get. At first I was in a wheelchair, wore a hard plastic waistcoat and only gradually began to walk using wooden crutches and a calliper on one leg. Kitty would push me into Youghal on my red-and-white tricycle and later back up a steep hill by a disused quarry filled with gorse. In the kitchen I rode around and around the table on my tricycle, swatting the flies hovering over it with a rolled-up newspaper. My right leg was not strong enough to push the pedal down so I had to use a hand to push my knee down to keep the tricycle moving. Emotionally I was more like a four- or five-year-old in my dependence on others and, with the egotism of a small child, I expected everybody to have nothing to do except look after me.

I am not sure how others perceived me. My cousin Shirley, whom I would have met in Myrtle Grove the day I fell ill if she had not gone for a walk with her nanny, spent the rest of the autumn confined to the grounds of the house. 'I was dreadfully upset when I saw you again,' she said. 'You were wearing callipers and my father carried you into the house and put you down on a sofa in the library.'[5]

Doctors believed that for two years after the illness it was possible through exercise to revive damaged muscles. Three times a week a hired car arrived at Brook Lodge and I lay down flat in the back seat. I became bored watching the tops of trees and buildings week after week from my prone position as we travelled the thirty miles to Cork. I would prod the driver in the back to encourage him to drive fast over hump-backed bridges so for an instant I had the satisfying sensation that the car had taken off before it bumped back on to the road. Once the driver turned to me in irritation and said: 'I think you are the most spoiled boy I have ever met.' In Cork we drove to City Hall, the large grey building by the Lee, where Pauline Kent, my physiotherapist, had a small cramped room upstairs. 'You try to find if there is a flicker of movement against gravity by the muscles,' she said. 'If there is you exercise these muscles to develop them and to stop the joints seizing up.'[6]

Pauline was energetic, able, short-tempered and over-worked. She found Dr Saunders patronising and unhelpful about her work. Once when he visited her, she snappishly asked: 'Why do I have to waste time walking a hundred yards to use a telephone and I don't even have a minute spare to go to the lavatory?' I liked her because she liked me and built up my determination to walk again. After a few months Pauline persuaded the Corporation to take over an old Turkish baths, a red-brick building in Cork's South Mall. I used to swim slowly in the pool with my legs trailing uselessly behind me.

I was taken to Whitechapel hospital in London for a series of operations on my feet, the purpose of which was to transfer the muscles, which had survived, to do the work of those that had died. By good fortune this type of operation had been pioneered by the brother of Kitty Muggeridge, the wife of Malcolm. My legs were covered in plaster casts and itched mercilessly. Malcolm gave me a long thin Moroccan dagger to scratch inside the plaster. He was a kindly figure, very tall like my father, whose smile illuminated his entire face like Mr Punch come to life. We stayed after the first operation with the Muggeridges at Robertsbridge in Sussex. I had learned how to play chess and he organised a chess tournament for me with Kingsley Martin, the editor of the *New Statesman*, my father and other friends.

I stopped using the plastic waistcoat and the wheelchair. Most important, my mother taught me to read through a form of gin-rummy combined with poker in which the players scored by inventing short words. I read nineteenth-century books for boys, particularly G. H. Henty and Robert Louis Stevenson, the lives of whose heroes did not seem dissimilar from those of my relatives. I spent hours vainly trying to throw one of my old-fashioned wooden crutches just like Long John Silver, as portrayed in a full-colour illustration in *Treasure Island*. Silver was shown striking a sailor, who refused to join his mutiny, in the back with a crutch hurled from fifteen feet away and killing him. Stevenson can never have tried using a crutch as a missile because I found that whatever I did the weight of the top of the crutch made it turn over and over in the air and rendered it ineffective as a weapon.

My parents must have recognised that I was becoming over-dependent on them. For all their political radicalism, they had rather traditional ideas about education. They may also have thought I was becoming 'spoiled' and too reliant on others. When I was nine they sent me as a day boy to St Stephen's School in Dublin, where Andrew was already a boarder. During my first term they rented a grim house with a dreary privet hedge in the Rathmines district so I could settle in, and afterwards I became a boarder myself. I did not enjoy exchanging life in a country house, where I was cosseted by parents and servants, for the dull routine of a schoolboy sleeping in a crowded dormitory. I did not like St Stephen's very much, but I did not hate it either. I was not well-educated in any traditional sense but I was well-read, highly competitive and liked to pass exams. I still used crutches until one day I threw them away and left them lying on a lawn behind the main schoolhouse. I could walk well enough without them and I was keen, with the conformity of a ten-year-old, to behave in the same way as the other boys. I could not play games so I spent most of my time reading. Academic pressure was not intense. The headmaster was the Reverend Hugh Brodie, the amiable former naval chaplain, who used to give us little pep talks before exams distinctly different in tone from that given by most schoolteachers. He would tell us that he himself had performed dismally in all the exams he had ever taken, but he had found that this made absolutely no difference to his life, which had on the whole been extremely enjoyable. Less amiable was the way in which he had sent Andrew to the railway station and not a hospital, though he must have guessed he had polio.

I was aware from an early age that I carried a lot of emotional scar tissue from polio. But I also – probably rightly – thought there was not much I could do about it. I spent a lot of time reading by myself, but I was not solitary and made friends easily. This was true at St Stephen's and later at Glenalmond, the public school built out of dark pink sandstone in Perthshire on the edge of the highland line to which I was dispatched at the age of thirteen. My father was right about the Scottish attitude

238

to education being more serious than in England. The school, established by Gladstone as an Anglican outpost amid the Scottish Presbyterians, was built on a bluff above a burn, an isolated but beautiful place. The barbarities of English school life were largely absent. This was thanks to more civilised Scottish traditions in education reinforced by the fact that many of the boys were the sons of lawyers from Edinburgh, litigious even by American standards, and capable of retaliating with a hail of writs against any suspected mistreatment of their offspring.

The nearest centre of civilisation to Glenalmond was Perth, a city which guidebooks at the time bleakly noted was 'known for its tea shops'. This was not an exciting prospect for a growing boy. At school I was social but I felt a certain remoteness, a gulf between myself and other people which was my fault rather than theirs. I remember Robin McMillan, a friend in my house at Glenalmond, later famous as an actor under the name of Robbie Coltrane, once saying to me in perplexity: 'You are a funny kind of introverted extrovert.' His father, a police doctor from Glasgow, used to take us out to lunch in Perth. He was dismissive of traffic regulations, possibly because he knew every policeman in Scotland. He would take short cuts by driving rapidly down one-way streets the wrong way. A kindly and humorous man, he regarded his patients with amused tolerance and took a certain proprietorial pride in the toughness of Glaswegians. He told me that one night he had been summoned to a stabbing in the city. He found the victim lying on the pavement with severe knife wounds to his stomach. Looking down on him was a plump man, clearly the attacker, with blood on his hands. 'Why did you do

239

it?' Dr McMillan asked him. 'He called me Fatty,' said the man with the air of one providing a satisfactory explanation.

I was eager to escape Glenalmond and I discovered that if you took a special Oxford entrance exam and were accepted they were not very interested in what marks you got at A levels. I was told this only a couple of days before the closing date for applications, without knowing much about Oxford or having seen it or any other university. I applied for Trinity College, which I had heard of because I had read a book about Bertrand Russell. It was only after I was accepted that somebody pointed out to me that Russell had gone to Trinity College, Cambridge. The only other college I knew about in Oxford was Christ Church, but for several years I had viewed the place with suspicion, because of a story told to me by Michael Flanders, my brother-in-law. He was the only person I knew well who had also caught polio and been badly crippled by it. A wheelchair was almost his trademark since he had achieved great success as a singer together with Donald Swann, producing best-selling records such as *A Drop of a Hat*. I think of him now as a bear of a man, but to a fourteen-year-old he was a friendly bear. His black beard reminded me of Captain Haddock in the Tintin stories. He married my half-sister Claudia, the daughter from my father's first marriage (he married three times), in 1959. Michael had been in his first year at Christ Church when he was called up and joined the navy. In 1943 he began to feel flu-like symptoms, but his commanding officer persuaded him to continue a voyage. By the time polio was diagnosed the virus had terribly damaged his legs, his back and one arm. He was left with only one lung. He could just walk with callipers and crutches but seldom did so, possibly because he found them demeaning. He lived most of his life in a wheelchair, though he could drive, which he did at great speed.[7]

Michael told me about Christ Church's brutal response to the disability of their former student. After being invalided out of the navy and spending time in hospital on an iron lung, he had applied to Christ Church to ask if he could return. He mentioned in a letter that he would need a ground-floor room and a small ramp so he could get his wheelchair up the steps. Christ Church wrote back promptly saying it was a university college, not a hospital, and could not accommodate him. He never returned. Years later, having achieved fame and fortune as a singer, Michael received a letter from Christ Church asking in unctuous terms if he would care to come back to his old college for some celebration. The writer said he was aware that Michael was confined to a wheelchair, but that suitable arrangements could easily be made for him to reach his room. Michael, who did not have a forgiving nature when it came to such snubs, described with glee the angry and contemptuous reply he had written, explaining why he would never again enter Christ Church in his life.

Michael's disability was severe because he was an adult when he caught the disease, a fact which frequently led to greater damage to the muscles. Worse still, he was leading a strenuous life at sea long after he was infected and before he was diagnosed. By the time the doctors did realise he had polio he could only be saved by being placed in an iron lung. If he had caught polio twenty years earlier he would probably have died because this sinister machine, which looked like a metal coffin, was only invented by an American engineer in 1928 in a bid to prevent children suffocating as their lungs failed.[8] It was effective and saved many lives, but it was a frightening symbol of how quickly the polio virus could bring its victims to the edge of death. Over the years, treatment of the illness had much improved but, for all their efforts, doctors in Britain or Ireland were not able to do much when Michael caught it during the Second World War or even when I was hit by the virus thirteen years later.

This was surprising since so many diseases were brought under control in the first half of the twentieth century. The polio virus was first identified during an epidemic in Vienna in 1908 and at first there was optimism that a cure would be swiftly found. But polio, as I have mentioned, was at home in the modern world where clean water and sanitation were robbing communities of natural immunity. The cities and countries which suffered epidemics were among the most prosperous and medically advanced places on earth: the USA, Sweden, Australia, Canada and Denmark. Early hopes of an effective vaccine were mocked by the rising number of victims during the summer months year after year. The worst polio epidemic in history was in the US in 1952 when there were 58,000 cases, 21,000 of whom were paralysed and more than 3,000 of whom died.[9]

I knew a few years after 1956 that a vaccine had been discovered which would have prevented me catching the disease. I did not think about it very much though I felt a little unlucky. I wondered whether my parents could have had me vaccinated in time, or whether I would have escaped illness had I been brought up in a country other than Ireland. In fact, there was little Claud and Patricia could have done unless they had taken the threat more seriously, and had had good medical contacts. My brother-in-law Nigel Murray, then at boarding school at Stowe, remembered getting a surprise summons from his father, a celebrated doctor, to meet him. His father drove him some distance down a road and then stopped the car, took a hypodermic out of its case and gave Nigel a painful injection of the Salk vaccine which he had just obtained. Church bells had famously rung out across America on 12 April 1955 to greet the first announcement of the successful mass field test of the vaccine invented by Jonas Salk. But it took time for vaccination programmes to be implemented and a faulty batch of vaccine, which actually gave polio to several hundred children, briefly dented public confidence. It was only over the next couple of years that mass inoculations began.

The conquest of polio was, nevertheless, one of the great American achievements of the twentieth century and was seen as such at the time. In terms of national prestige it was the medical equivalent of the landing on the moon. The peculiar nature of the disease made it easier to attract popular attention than it would have been with other illnesses. Polio terrified people because it struck randomly at their children. There seemed no way of avoiding it. It not only affected the rich as well as the poor, but the better-off were more likely to catch it because of their lack of immunity. It paralysed President Roosevelt below the waist when he caught it in 1920. It was FDR's lawyer Basil O'Connor who organised the National Foundation for Infantile Paralysis and the so-called March of Dimes, the collection of money from every house and high street in America. The battle against polio had a feeling of common endeavour seldom seen outside wartime. Polio was easy to publicise because it produced such frightening images. In posters and on film, crutches, callipers and wheelchairs were shown preying on smiling children. The sheer quantity of money available had a positive impact. Jonas Salk, the scientist whose inactivated or 'killed' virus was the first effective vaccine, only undertook polio research at first because it was the sole means by which he could obtain funding for his laboratory in Pittsburgh.

Cork was not the only city in the world where there was a polio epidemic in 1956. Some weeks before the first cases were reported in Ireland, it had also begun to spread in Chicago. The response in the two cities was very different. By the end of August there had been 880 cases and twenty-five deaths in Chicago.[10] The result was that Chicago became one of the first cities in America to start using the Salk vaccine as soon as it was pronounced safe. It had suffered an epidemic in 1952 with 1,203 cases of polio of whom eighty-two died. There had been a well-organised but ineffective campaign to stop the spread of the illness by closing beaches, cinemas and swimming pools as well as eradicating rodents and insects. It had not been enough. In early 1956 the rising number of cases of polio in Chicago suggested that a second epidemic was on its way. This time health workers took action to stop it in its tracks by mass inoculation. They took over vacant stores, garage forecourts, street corners, parks and the backs of trucks to give injections. September and October were supposed to be the worst months for polio but by the end of August the disease was under control and the number of new victims began to fall.

In Britain the official medical attitude to polio was more phlegmatic, not to say uncaring, than in the US. When it did spread, the first instinct of British doctors, as in Ireland a few years later, was to play down what was happening under the pretence that this was necessary to prevent a mass panic. The first epidemic in Britain was in 1947 when the number of cases jumped to 7,776, having previously never exceeded 1,500 a year. An editorial in the *British Medical Journal* is almost a caricature of supine evasiveness:

A state of panic is rather easily produced by Press publicity, and it is to be hoped that the daily newspapers in this country will not draw undue attention to the present outbreak. In any year the cases and deaths due to poliomyelitis will be far fewer than the injuries and deaths caused by road accidents.[11]

The European countries which were quickest to use the new vaccine were in Scandinavia. Sweden had been ravaged by the disease; it was the country's fifth-largest killer of young children.[12] Denmark too was badly hit: one of the worst polio epidemics ever took place in Copenhagen in 1952 where victims asphyxiated because there was only a single iron lung in the main hospital. The Danes rapidly improvised, keeping people breathing by hand, using relays of medical students. Four years later the same system was adopted in Cork.

At the time that Andrew and I caught polio most of the mysteries about the disease had been penetrated by scientists. Over the previous decade they had learned about how the virus infected its victims and in a few cases crippled their bodies. But I don't think any of my family had much idea of how polio operated. We had been influenced a little here by the Victorian feeling that it was chicken-hearted to think too much about one's own health. Our ignorance, however, is surprising since my family were obsessive readers of newspapers and the doctors in Cork spelled out, though without much effect, that it was difficult not to be infected whatever precautions were taken. They also implied that it was the better-off and most isolated who would be the most vulnerable.

Thirteen

For most of the year the west wind blew out of the Atlantic into Youghal bay. The town with its ancient quays had been built on the east side of a steep hill to protect it from storms. In February the fishermen in their small boats put to sea to fish for salmon. But in early 1956 the wind blew steadily and unexpectedly from the east for week after week. 'There were no fish,' recalled Paddy Linehan, the owner of the Moby Dick pub overlooking a quay where fishing boats tied up to the bollards. 'The wind blew from the east for six weeks so the fishermen couldn't catch salmon and soon they were all dependent on the St Vincent de Paul [Society].'[1] The fishermen were among the poorest people in Youghal in the middle of the 1950s, but there were others living on the edge of destitution. After a brief post-war boom the economy was stagnant. Mass emigration soared. In 1957 an Irish-American academic named John Kelleher even suggested that the Irish might, going by current trends, be about to vanish from history.[2] As a child I found nothing strange about the fact that I never saw any buildings under construction, but in almost every

247

field there were ruined cottages and houses fading into the landscape as they were engulfed by the exuberant Irish vegetation.

The Irish economic revival is usually placed at the end of the 1950s but in Youghal there were earlier signs of it. Mr John Murray's carpet factory was set up in old eighteenth-century warehouses near the quays in 1954. 'It grew like topsy,' said Paddy Linehan who, as a member of the local council, had spent years seeking to attract industry to the town. 'It grew and grew and grew until there were eight hundred men there. They were selling the carpets to hotels in Las Vegas.' This was still in the future, but already the horses, gigs, carts and traps, providing enough work for two blacksmiths, were starting to disappear from the narrow main street. Ireland had not truly been part of the Third World since the beginning of the century. It was peaceful. There was little crime. It had a competent civil service. The health system had limited resources but worked. There was universal education. If it was stagnant it was also stable. John Gowen, the doctor who looked after my family, set up his practice in Youghal in the late 1940s. He said: 'There was no shortage of food though there was of clothing. Nothing much had changed in 150 years. The worst epidemic disease was TB.'[3]

Not that these achievements were entirely a matter for self-congratulation because so many Irish problems were exported. People responded to poverty and unemployment by voting with their feet. In the years 1951 to 1956 net emigration was 197,000 from a country with a population of only about three million. In the next five years it was 212,000.[4] The last owner of Brook Lodge, who refused to sell it to my parents, was an Irish-American policeman in Los Angeles. He had inherited it from his father, the old man whom my parents had found living in one room below a giant crucifix, just at the moment that we rented it. The new owner would not sell because, like many Irish emigrants, he was always planning to return to Ireland but never did so.

Many explanations were given half a century later as to why Ireland became so prosperous. By 2004 East European countries joining the European Union were studying the Irish experience to see if they could repeat it. Historians began to trace back early signs of modern development. Never mentioned, not surprisingly, is the polio epidemic in Cork, though it was a clear sign that Ireland in the 1950s had more in common with New York than it did with Nairobi. This may not have been obvious to fishermen in Youghal in the spring of 1956, compelled to live on charity because of the dearth of salmon. But a few months later Cork was to join a select group of modern and wealthy cities – Chicago, Los Angeles, New York, Copenhagen and Stockholm – hit by polio epidemics during the twentieth century. The reasons for this were well known to local doctors at the time and were frequently reported in the press, but this made little dent in the popular perception that polio and poverty were linked. In reality, as we have seen, it was the growing lack of natural immunity because of clean-water supply and modern sewerage systems which made these cities vulnerable.

Polio was little noticed in Ireland until 1942. It was not even a notifiable disease and no figures on the numbers of cases were collected. When Pauline Kent's sister caught bulbar polio, the most lethal variant of the disease which affects the brain stem, in the 1930s, the family doctor near Fermoy at first diagnosed encephalitis and then meningitis. She had complained of a headache on Christmas Eve and died on 28 December.[5] There were advantages, as my father pointed out to me, in catching polio during an epidemic when doctors were generally alert for the symptoms which could so easily be mistaken for flu or a minor ailment. Though even at the height of the epidemic in Cork one man who had caught polio was told by a doctor that he was suffering from a slipped disc.[6] The first real epidemic in Ireland was in 1942–43 when there were 487 cases and 133 deaths which meant a death rate of 27.4 per cent.[7] It had begun in Dublin when sixty-four people were treated at the Cork Street hospital. The disease became more common. There was an outbreak in Londonderry in 1953. In the same year there were rumours of an epidemic in Cork but the Chief Medical Officer said later that there had been only one minor case.[8]

Dr Saunders had a clear idea about why the city was becoming vulnerable. He explained that for centuries people had been living in happy symbiosis with polio until this was disturbed by improved standards of living. He had read the 'First Report of the Expert Committee on Poliomyelitis', established by the World Health Organisation in Rome in 1955. The report said:

In general, it would seem that the poorer the standard of living and sanitation of a people, the more extensively is poliomyelitis virus disseminated among them and the lower is the apparent incidence of paralytic poliomyelitis . . . It is of considerable significance that widespread epidemics first occurred in Scandinavia, the northern USA, Australia and New Zealand.

The WHO expected other countries, as their standard of living rose, also to suffer epidemics.[9] Communities attacked once by the polio virus were often revisited every three years. The epidemic broke out in the summer, with September and October proving the worst months. Even in relatively modern cities the level of natural immunity was often quite high. A survey in Belfast in 1956 showed that 70 per cent of the children were immune, though the figure was expected to be lower in the countryside.[10]

The number of people crippled or killed by the polio virus was small in Ireland, as it was in the rest of the world, compared to the number of victims of tuberculosis. The degree of fear created by the disease was out of proportion to the number of casualties. People were terrified by the possibility that their children might be crippled. The Irish were perhaps more conscious of the illness than the British, because its effects were so highly publicised in the US and most Irish people had Irish-American relatives. There had been few cases of polio in Youghal before Andrew and I got it, but the sufferings of those crippled by it were well known in town. Just before Christmas 1953 Maura McGuane, a seventeen-year-old schoolgirl at the Loreto convent, felt a pain in her legs which became weaker by the day. Her parents were drapers and had a shop in town. 'It was a bad age to get it,' she said. 'It was the moment you should be breaking out into the world. I missed *Moby Dick* in 1954.'

She spent two years in St Finbarr's. A cheerful intelligent woman who came to live in Church Street near Kitty Lee, Maura worried about whether she would fit in again once she was out, since she could only move with callipers or in a wheelchair. 'You think that life is over,' she said. 'I knew things would not get any better.' Later she added thoughtfully that she had 'never been unhappy'.[11]

The impact of polio depended on the personality and age of the victim. Peggy Brennan from Mitchelstown was a child when she caught it in 1941 and was taken to the Mercy hospital. Her legs were badly affected. She says: 'In childhood you don't see your own disabilities.' I am not sure this is entirely true, but it is true that as a child the effect of the disabilities is more closely integrated, for good or ill, into one's identity. For the older victims the effect is more shocking. People who can walk and run and direct their own lives without being dependent on anyone else, can suddenly find themselves, like my brother-in-law Michael Flanders, permanently confined to a wheelchair and reliant on others helping them. Donal Walsh, a farmer from just outside Blarney, got the disease in October 1957 when he was twenty-two. Crippled in the legs and back, he told me how he 'cried bitterly when I realised what had happened to me'. Later he was 'terrified of coming home. I didn't know if they would understand my disability.' All three of these people, like myself, came from strong and comparatively well-off families. For the poorer victims, whose families had neither the time nor the resources to look after them, the outlook was altogether more grim. 'Some people are bitter,' reflects Donal

Walsh. 'They felt they have been dealt a poor hand in life, especially if they never got married.'[12]

In 1955, a year before the start of the epidemic in Cork, the Department of Health in Dublin had a strong suspicion that there was going to be an onslaught of the disease. It knew that figures for polio cases had risen sharply every three years and the previous peaks had been in 1947, 1950 and 1953, with a trough in the two years in between. They rightly believed it was likely to recur in 1956. The reason for the three-year cycle was probably that, while the number of cases officially notified in these years were in each case still less than three hundred, they only represented the tip of the iceberg. Tens of thousands of others had got polio without knowing it. The pool of people susceptible to the virus fell and it took two years for it to be replenished.[13]

The Department of Health did not spell out why it suspected that Ireland would soon see a surge in the number of polio cases. It sent out a carefully written three-page letter to county officials and health officers around Ireland telling them in detail how to respond in the event of an outbreak. It admitted that control of an epidemic would be difficult because 'for each paralytic case there are many other unrecognised cases'. In other words there would be many carriers of the disease who showed no symptoms but could give it to anybody they met. The identity of these carriers would be impossible to determine. Nevertheless, some methods of control were important. Doctors had to be able to diagnose the disease accurately and quickly. Once a person was diagnosed all 'family contacts, especially children, should be regarded as probably infected with the virus'. Everybody should avoid physical exertion and should not handle foodstuffs to be consumed by people outside the family circle. Children must be kept at home for twenty-one days. Anybody who felt ill should go to bed and call a doctor.

The Department of Health clearly understood that the virus entered the body through the mouth and was extruded in shit. Among the ten measures recommended in order to avoid infection was frequent washing of the hands after going to the lavatory and before meals. Food should be protected from flies and use of common towels avoided.[14] There was some evidence that these simple rules did have an effect. A year earlier in 1954, Queen Elizabeth II was due to visit Western Australia where an epidemic had just started. The authorities wondered if they should ban children from attending the festivities because this might spread the disease. Instead they decided that every child must carefully wash his or her hands after going to the toilet. This seems to have worked. Not only was there no increase in children catching polio but the number fell during and immediately after the Queen's visit.[15]

Some suggestions by the Department caused trouble later. It was easy for everybody to agree that unchlorinated swimming baths should be closed. It had also suggested that immunisation schemes against other diseases be stopped, as well as operations to remove tonsils or teeth. None of these measures was controversial. But, as we have seen, others, such as discouraging 'unnecessary travel into, or out of, communities where the disease is prevalent', could spell the ruin of local business. There were also sharp divisions over the closure of schools. The Department left this to the local Chief Medical Officer but advised reopening them if they were already closed for the holidays. The doctors in charge in Cork generally thought this was pointless as they were convinced that quarantine measures would never be rigorous enough to stop the illness. The intense and at times hysterical pressure for closing schools, cinemas and sports events all came from a frightened public and not from the doctors.

The system worked relatively well. The same day that I was taken to hospital a man arrived at 10 p.m. at the house of Dick Cunningham, a friendly farmer with three hundred acres whose farmhouse was a field away from Brook Lodge. He was our closest neighbour and once he had shown me how to milk one of his cows. I had been playing with one of his daughters a few days before. The late-night visitor explained that he was from the Department of Health and added: 'I have bad news.' He said that I had just been sent to St Finbarr's with suspected polio. The Cunninghams were asked to keep their children at home for several weeks. It did not have much effect on their lives, but other farmers were not so lucky. Many of them drew part of their small income from milk. Every few hundred yards on country roads at this time there were concrete plinths where milk churns were left for collection by lorries. But if one member of a farmer's family was known to have caught polio then the milk-lorry drivers would refuse to collect the churns. 'The ones you really felt sorry for were the farming children,' recalls Dr O'Callaghan. 'Nobody wanted their milk and they depended on the milk cheque. It was extraordinary how people shunned them.'[16]

The belief that milk was infected by the virus may have been the unintended result of a prolonged campaign by the powerful Irish farming lobby against the pasteurisation of milk. The government had been trying to introduce legislation to reduce the danger from milk since the 1920s when Ireland, together with Hungary, had the highest incidence of non-pulmonary and bovine tuberculosis in Europe. Just before the First World War a British official had described the Irish as 'our great reservoir of consumption'.[17] When pasteurised milk was finally introduced it was regarded with suspicion. During the first days of the epidemic in Cork a rumour spread that the polio virus was being transmitted through the milk. To stop the panic, a statement was issued by Dr Saunders and Dr R. J. Cussen, the Chief Veterinary Officer. It said firmly:

> We desire to state emphatically that there is not a vestige of truth in this suggestion. We are investigating at present the complaints in regard to the souring of pasteurised milk. All that can be said at this juncture is that from experiments carried out by us personally and from enquiries made by a number of reputable persons, pasteurised milk has stood up to every test imposed and has remained fresh and sweet for periods of thirty-six hours or more.

Even so, Saunders tried not to be too dismissive of people's fears by suggesting that they examine the seals of bottles of pasteurised milk to see if they had been tampered with.[18]

Overall, little more could be done in 1956 to arrest the disease once it had been caught than could have been for the infant Sir Walter Scott when he caught it in 1773.[19] Almost two hundred years later it was possible to keep victims alive through the iron lung. Operations on the feet could help restore mobility. But there were still severe limits on what doctors and physiotherapists could do, even with limitless resources. Of course, resources in Ireland *were* limited, but after 1953, when there were 245 cases of polio and thirty-three deaths, the Department of Health began to reorganise in order to meet the threat. Its officials knew that other countries had achieved good results by concentrating experienced doctors, nurses and special equipment in special treatment centres. Here patients were treated when they still had the fever. Three regional poliomyelitis centres were set up, at St Finbarr's in Cork, at the Dublin Fever hospital and at the Galway Regional hospital. There were also two 'respiratory first aid centres' established in Sligo and Donegal to keep people breathing and alive until they could be brought to a bigger hospital. The Department of Health sought the advice of the Medical Research Council of Ireland on the advances in vaccination in the US, and started a survey on the degree of natural immunity among children in different parts of the country. Its results, which showed that natural immunity was limited, were overtaken by the 1956 epidemic.

St Finbarr's seemed to have very basic facilities when I was in it, but it was a lot better than anything that had existed before. Since the Second World War Dr Goold, the Resident Medical Supervisor, had been building it up. St Mary's hospital at Gurranebraher had been under construction for years and was originally designed as a sanatorium for TB patients. It was divided up into isolated separate buildings, each with two wards. But in 1955 it was still being equipped and at the last minute was turned into an orthopaedic hospital for polio victims. Anne

O'Sullivan, who had just qualified as a nurse, arrived at the hospital early in 1956. She said: 'At this time things weren't great. The equipment wasn't there.'[20] The hospital had an authoritarian system, with the senior doctors wholly in charge. John Hall, starting off as a medical student in 1956, thought: 'The quality of the nursing depended very much on the quality of the sisters in charge. Some were strong disciplinarians and others were mediocre.'[21]

With children who had polio and were still infectious, there was a reason for not allowing their parents to visit them in the wards. But overall family members were excluded as far as possible. 'I could never fathom it,' said Hall. 'Children had to accept total isolation from the family when they were ill. It was an extraordinary thing. I would always let parents come to the door.' He thought there was something here of the attitude of the old Health Boards dealing with paupers who had nowhere else to go. St Finbarr's had been built as a workhouse after the Famine and its inmates then had included unmarried mothers and vagrants. My father had the same impression as Professor Hall when he visited me at Gurranebraher, though he mistakenly thought that the other patients were all very poor. He said:

I had the impression that the hospital people, aware of this extreme poverty, subconsciously treated it as a partial excuse for the failure to give the unhappy children the kind of psychological amenities they should have had. It was felt that they were lucky to have a fine room and good food.[22]

*

It was never clear why polio could strike so devastatingly in one city or district and find no victims next door. Though the subject of extensive research, some of the mysteries about the operation of the disease have never been cleared up. In general terms it is easy to define the targets of the virus. As previously stated, in its epidemic form polio commonly struck at people in modern cities and with permanent access to clean water and sewage disposal. But such generalisations about polio can be a little deceptive. The first well-known epidemic in the US in 1894 was not in a city but in Rutland County in rural Vermont where a hundred children were paralysed. A study by the US Public Health Service of 200,000 families in 1935 showed that poverty and insanitary living conditions did not necessarily protect people against the disease. The worst epidemic in the Netherlands was in 1943 during the German occupation when food supplies and public hygiene were poor. Another epidemic took place in Berlin in 1947 when many of its inhabitants were living amid the ruins. It may be, of course, that in Amsterdam and Berlin the inhabitants had lost their immunity during prosperous pre-war days and were peculiarly vulnerable when these ended. The early history of polio may also be distorted by lack of information or recognition of the disease. It is possible that small unexplained epidemics had been taking place in rural areas for centuries but had not been recorded.[23] The outbreak of polio among the children of St Helena in the first half of the nineteenth century is only well known because Charles Bell, the famous Scottish doctor, was consulted several years later by the mother of one of the crippled children on the island and he afterwards mentioned what had happened in a lecture in 1844.[24]

Other factors had to be at work as well as lack of immunity, though they might be affected by it. The number of polio cases in the US increased sharply in 1942, possibly because in the first year of American involvement in the war young men from country districts, lacking the appropriate antibodies, were called up as soldiers and were coming into contact with the virus for the first time. In poor and unhygienic households you were more likely to be protected against the virus but you were also more likely to meet it. The precise ingredients which went into creating a polio epidemic remain uncertain. It is also not known why one person should be paralysed out of every hundred or two hundred people infected. The virulence and quantity of the virus played a role, as did the extent to which the victim remained active after he caught polio.

In Cork the spread of polio in 1956 showed none of these peculiarities. It was very much a classic epidemic. It came, as expected, three years after the last peak of polio cases in Ireland and in a city where there had been little polio before. The doctors were quick to identify the districts worst affected. At this time Cork still had horrendous slums. John Hall remembers visiting tenements in the north of the city 'where there was no furniture in the rooms and no men also. They were all working as builders' labourers repairing bomb damage in England.'[25] But it was not here that polio was most widespread. On 10 August Dr Saunders completed a report on the epidemic based on what he had seen. He wrote: 'The regions most heavily affected are those in which housing and general sanitation have reached their highest development – Ballyphehane, Killeenreendowney, Gurranebraher, Churchfield, Spangle

Hill.'[26] Everybody else coping with the epidemic similarly noticed that it was the better-off who were being hardest hit. Other witnesses – doctors, nurses, officials – all make the same point when recollecting the epidemic fifty years later, speaking as if it was a fact which had surprised them. Their expectation of the behaviour of killer diseases was based on their experiences with typhoid, cholera, dysentery and typhus. In Cork most of the victims were in the relatively prosperous southern suburbs and not in the terrible slums in the north of the city. Dr Gerald McCarthy, the Medical Officer for the county, pointed this out, saying: 'The higher the standard of living the greater tendency towards the disease. Generally the well-washed and the well-laundered children are the most susceptible.'[27] Maureen O'Sullivan, the Red Cross nurse who took her ambulance into every part of the city, noticed that '80 per cent of the victims came from affluent or semi-affluent families'.[28]

The epidemic which was about to start had one peculiarity: it began earlier than was normal. Epidemics all over the world invariably broke out in the summer months, but in the past in Europe had usually reached their peak in September and October.[29] The rule was not invariable. In the US a study had shown that polio cases peaked four weeks earlier in the southern states than in the north, on 15 August where the peak in the north was on 15 September.[30] Possibly the early outbreak of the disease is explained by the fact that the summer of 1956 was long remembered in Ireland not only for the polio epidemic but for the fact that it was extremely hot. Instead of the uncertain Irish weather, the bane of the tourist trade, the sun shone down for day after day.

At the start of the summer there were already some patients in the polio ward in St Finbarr's. The first to arrive in March was a man called Michael O'Connor from Stradbally. He was a farmer's son, a buyer for the local leather factory, aged about thirty-three, six foot one in height, good-looking and a keen sportsman and fisherman. He had been to a conference in Dublin and on his return came down with a heavy flu. His wife called a doctor and an ambulance took him to Cork. What happened next helps explain why polio so terrified people. He lost all movement in his limbs, both legs and arms. He never breathed naturally again. He was placed on a 'Beaver', the variant of the iron lung, which blew air into his lungs through a hole cut in his throat. His sister Mary recalls that his mind remained sharp and he could read, but members of the family had to turn the pages of his book. He remained totally immobile, except when a nurse moved him, for nine and a half years 'until he wasted away and died'.[31] The next victim was a six-year-old boy from Tralee in Kerry.[32] But both these cases came from far outside Cork city and probably had nothing to do with the approaching epidemic.

The first polio victim in Cork was diagnosed on 13 June. Six days later there were another two cases. This was worrying, but still not abnormal for the summer months. But by 3 July the number of people with polio had risen to six. Dr Saunders concluded: 'Since this was equal to the maximum number of cases occurring previously in any one year, it was deemed that an epidemic was imminent.'[33] On 7 July there was an article in the

Cork Examiner, very deliberately not leading the front page, announcing: 'CORK CITY POLIO OUTBREAK: SIX CASES'. The sub-heading told readers: 'NO OCCASION FOR UNDUE ALARM – MEDICAL OFFICER'. It soon became clear that people in Cork were not only unduly alarmed but were beginning to panic. It was at this stage that the rumour spread that pasteurised milk was responsible for the outbreak. Reports of the epidemic had already started to circulate from 5 July. The Victoria Swimming Baths were closed and Dr Saunders warned that it was dangerous to swim in any part of the River Lee which flows through Cork. On 9 July, after three more suspected cases of polio were diagnosed, Dr Saunders called on parents to 'get your children to bed before nightfall and help to stop the possible spread of the disease'.[34] The link between polio and swimming, though it is certainly one of many ways of catching the disease, seems to have been an obsession in Cork. Cork Corporation considered at a meeting on 10 July if it could prosecute people for swimming in the Lee near the Opera House. They were described as 'a danger to themselves and to others whom they contacted'. The following day was considered particularly bad because of another increase in the number reporting sick. A visit of Buff Bill's circus to the city was cancelled at short notice at the request of Dr Saunders. He said: 'I put the facts before them and they cooperated to the full extent, in spite of the obvious financial loss involved.'[35]

By the middle of the month there had been twenty-five confirmed cases of polio taken to St Finbarr's. Even the *Cork Examiner* admitted that polio was 'rampant in Cork City'. A young girl who had been admitted the previous day had just died of bulbar polio. So far the doctors noted with relief that most victims were suffering from the milder Brunhilde or Type 1 of the three main types of polio, though people in Cork understandably saw this as being less than reassuring. In terms of impact it was as if parents of a later generation had been told that their children might contract Aids but it was of a mild form, more likely to cripple than to kill. Dr Goold was forced to publicly deny a rumour that 'there were many more cases of polio apart from those announced'.[36]

The number of people being admitted to St Finbarr's rose inexorably to forty-two confirmed cases by 20 July. Sean O'Casey, the Lord Mayor, walked around the city to see how people were responding to warnings that children should go to bed early, wash their hands regularly, avoid contact with other children and not exert themselves. O'Casey said he was 'dismayed and disappointed to find children playing on the streets at a very late hour'. Fear of meeting anybody from Cork who might be carrying the virus was beginning to spread. British naval patrol vessels berthed at the quays in Cork refused to allow anybody to visit them.[37] Commercial travellers from Cork found that their customers in other parts of the country showed a sudden enthusiasm for discussing business on the phone and avoided personal interviews.[38] Churches held Masses with prayers that the disease should not spread further. It was also beginning to be noticed that even in a city as small as Cork not all districts were equally affected. Most victims came from the south side of the city, sometimes from new suburbs, like Douglas, that were not yet within the city boundaries as well as two districts in the county, Lombardstown and Buttevant, in north Cork.

In the third week of the month the epidemic was still gathering strength. On 23 July nine new cases were admitted to St Finbarr's bringing the total to fifty-five confirmed cases and twelve suspected. Dr Goold told the South Cork Board of Public Assistance, the body in overall charge of St Finbarr's, that there 'is a panic reaction to the polio epidemic in Cork, which is totally without justification and there must be an intelligent approach to it'.[39] The local politicians he was addressing did not find this reassuring. They asked about the possibility of vaccination and Dr Goold told them that experiments with the vaccine were being carried out in Britain but not during the summer months (this was because it was feared that injections might help spread the disease). No doubt Dr Goold thought he was reducing the intense anxiety of his troubled audience, but even at this distance in time his words are strikingly counter-productive.

Professionals in any crisis deeply affecting the public must deal with the same dilemma as that facing Dr Goold, who had no experience in coping with such a disaster. They must take every measure to avert or alleviate the emergency. This means proceeding as if the worst-case scenario was inevitable by acting in good time to avert exactly such a dire outcome. But at the same time people in responsible positions want to avoid mass panic by continually asserting that things are not as bad as they look and they have everything under control. In Dublin, health officials were getting themselves into a twist by simultaneously telling people that it was perfectly safe to visit Cork, but at the same time saying they should not go there if they could possibly avoid it.

Before the end of the month more powerful guns were

brought out to reassure people in Cork. Dr Lucey, the Roman Catholic Bishop of Cork, a famously influential and vocal cleric, ordered a letter from himself to be read out in all churches and special prayers to be said on 28 July 'for the abatement of poliomyelitis and the good health of all stricken by it'. He reiterated that there was no reason to panic, the outbreak was mild and the local authorities had the situation under control. But Dr Lucey diplomatically underlined the real seriousness of the situation by writing: 'I ask those who have no children of their own to come to the Mass if they possibly can and join with the priest in this solemn act of intercession and Christian solidarity.' The unspoken message was that children, possibly infectious or vulnerable to infection if they congregated together, should not be brought to church.[40]

By now children were being sent out of the city by their parents to friends and relatives elsewhere in Ireland. On 27 July T. F. O'Higgins, the Minister of Health, came down from Dublin to attend a conference in City Hall of all those involved in dealing with the epidemic. He later toured St Finbarr's hospital and expressed himself highly satisfied with all he saw. Asked afterwards by reporters what he thought of the flight of children from Cork, he said that 'in view of the mildness of the epidemic he thought there was no need for public alarm and there should be no mass exodus from the city, nor should people wishing to visit the city hesitate to do so'. These were the usual encouraging noises expected of a general visiting the front line. But it was not the best day to make such optimistic pronouncements. While O'Higgins was speaking another ten suspected cases were brought to St Finbarr's, the highest number admitted so far on one day.

All were confirmed as having caught polio, bringing to eighty-three the total number of victims.[41] It was about now that my family and I sailed up the Lee into Cork on the *Innisfallen* and found the streets of the city so eerily deserted by its people.

Fourteen

I used to wonder in later years if I reacted more strongly than other children to catching polio and being confined in a hospital because I had been so carefully protected growing up in Brook Lodge. Either my mother or Kitty was always with me. It was the first time in my life that I had to cope with the world all by myself. It turned out, however, that I was not the only child who found Gurranebraher a brutal place and retreated into silent misery.

One of the first six victims of the disease, whose diagnosis convinced Dr Saunders that he was facing an epidemic, was a ten-year-old girl called Helena Casey. The daughter of a bus driver living in Ballinalough not far from St Finbarr's, she was diagnosed on 1 July as having caught polio. She hated the hospital. 'It was an awful place,' she recalls. 'I was in the children's ward which was very crowded and had three iron lungs in the middle of the room. The food was horrible. I was highly indignant because they put a rubber sheet on the bed in case I wet it.' Separated from her mother and father, she could only glimpse them through a diamond-shaped pane of glass in the window.

A few days later Helena's three-year-old sister Pat also fell ill. It was one of the myths in Cork before the epidemic that if one member of a family got polio the others would be spared. This was being rapidly disproved. 'I was put to bed in a boxroom upstairs,' says Pat. 'My mother brought me up a plate of potatoes and gravy. I immediately threw up and I remember my mother shouting to my father: "She's got it too."' She was in a high fever. An ambulance was called and Pat recalls her father frantically following it on his bicycle as it drove to St Finbarr's. For some unknown reason the doctors and nurses kept it a secret from Helena that her younger sister was also in the hospital. She only learned about it from overhearing two nurses talking and demanded to see Pat who was in a cot with high bars in another ward. A potty was put in her bed. Helena told a nurse: 'She'll never use it.' A nurse replied: 'She must.' Pat remembers the nurses as being 'terrible, absolutely horrible'.

The two sisters felt very isolated. One day Pat saw from a window her mother arrive at the hospital entrance with oranges and comics but they were never delivered. Helena, her legs badly weakened, was moved to Gurranebraher. Once there she discovered she was banned from sending letters home, 'so they were smuggled out by a cleaning lady who used to take my father's bus and hand them over to him'. This is difficult to understand since everybody who was moved from St Finbarr's to St Mary's at Gurranebraher was meant to be over the infectious phase of the disease. It may have been a hangover from the era when the hospital was intended for TB patients who would have been dangerously infectious. Helena recalls two nursing sisters, one tall and one short but fierce, as 'real dragons. We all hated them. It was like prisoners against the Nazis. But sometimes the night nurses would make us tea and toast and sing with us.'

The psychological impact of suddenly being cast into a hostile environment was harder to endure for the younger child. In the case of the Casey sisters it was the older girl, Helena, who suffered the worst long-term physical damage. But Pat, only three years old, stopped speaking as I was to do a few months later and refused to utter a word even when she was taken home. She reverted to behaving like a baby and would only take milk from a bottle. 'I didn't talk to anybody,' she said. 'I used to hide under the kitchen table when visitors came to the house because I thought they would take me back to the hospital.' The trauma was deep. Some twenty-two years later Pat had to go back to the hospital with a sick relative. By now the big ward where she had been so miserable had changed and was divided into cubicles. Even so, when Pat entered the lobby her old fears all revived and she had to hastily leave the building.[1]

Dr Goold at St Finbarr's and Dr St John O'Connell at Gurranebraher never seemed to realise what their younger patients were going through. The doctors in charge were, in any case, Olympian figures. In their visits to the wards they were like generals reviewing the troops and the ward sisters behaved like so many sergeant-majors. It was not a system likely to reveal how small and frightened children felt about their experience. Nor were the doctors likely to give priority to the psychological impact of the disease when they were trying to limit its physical effects. But they also had a difficulty in seeing the victims of polio as anything other than patients. Seeing suffering every day immunised them against it. Dr Goold complained irritably, even when infectious diseases were not involved, about the inconvenience to staff of families trying to visit their relatives.

The local press never named any of the people who had caught polio. This dehumanised the victims but the impact of the self-censorship exacerbated the sense of crisis. It created a vacuum of information about the epidemic, and the doctors should not have complained too much if it was filled with frightening rumours. August was expected to see the peak of the epidemic. By the end of the first week of the month the number of confirmed cases had risen to 113 with another four suspected.[2] But reports in the *Cork Examiner* and the *Evening Echo*, before television by far the most influential sources of information locally, became more and more like short military bulletins, accurate in so far as they went but very short on detail. Only official accounts of what was happening were published. Both papers developed a strong interest in foreign news. Conveniently for them many other exciting and important events were happening in the world. It was the year of the Hungarian uprising and the Suez crisis. At the same time as my family returned to Ireland in early August, Sir Anthony Eden was stressing the dependence of Britain on Middle East oil and concealing his secret agreement with France and Israel to overthrow Nasser. 'This is a matter of life and death to us all,' said Eden, justifying the invasion of Egypt in very similar words to those used half a century later by Tony Blair and President George W. Bush to justify the invasion of Iraq. 'Our quarrel is not with Egypt, still less with the Arab world. It is with Colonel Nasser.'[3] It was the ebb tide of the British Empire. British forces were fighting EOKA guerrillas in Cyprus in the same sort of war that they had been fighting in Cork thirty-five years earlier, and with equal lack of success.

The local papers were happy to write colourful and detailed stories, this time giving the names, about victims of polio so long as they were struck down far from Ireland. In the South Pacific, 140 miles from New Zealand, for instance, a Dr A. McFarland, a twenty-six-year-old doctor from Belfast, had been on his way to take up a medical appointment aboard the liner *Rangitoto* when he was found to have caught polio. There were three other victims on board. Dr McFarland had trouble breathing. A Bristol freighter plane flew over the *Rangitoto* and dropped breathing equipment. The crew was seen to pick it up from the sea. But five minutes later the New Zealand office of the shipping company which owned the *Rangitoto* received a radio message saying that Dr McFarland had just died. In Cork the doctors were doing their best to keep the figures for polio as low as possible. Those for the city and county were issued separately. Victims from Kerry and Waterford and other counties who were brought to St Finbarr's were not added to the total from Cork itself. On 10 August a six-year-old girl called Mary O'Sullivan from Mallow in north Cork died. Initially it was suspected that she was another victim of the epidemic, but Dr Goold announced with relief: 'Clinical and post-mortem findings definitely excluded the possibility that polio was the cause of death.'[4]

A year before the epidemic the Department of Health had said that in the event of an outbreak of polio travel in and out of the restricted area should be limited as far as possible. In as small a country as Ireland, with no natural boundaries, this was not easy to do. Some of the doctors in Cork were openly contemptuous of the idea. At the end of August Dr Gerald McCarthy wrote to the Department of Health: 'The restrictions being enjoined on Cork County residents are, in my opinion, unduly strict and in any case they are quite nonsensical while the C.I.E. [rail] line Cork–Kingsbridge and the Cork–Dublin highway via Naas are still open.'[5] But while an effective cordon sanitaire might be impractical there was no doubt, as we have seen, that people from the rest of Ireland were frightened of meeting anybody from Cork. A local Galway politician and member of the Dáil [the Irish parliament] called John Geoghegan angrily telephoned the office of T. F. O'Higgins on 8 August to say that people in Galway and nearby Salthill had been very perturbed to see 'an excursion train which went from Cork to Galway last Sunday with 250 people (including many children)'. He wanted an assurance that this would not happen again during the polio epidemic in Cork. Geoghegan must have been fully aware that there was not much a government minister could do to stop people from Cork travelling and simply wanted to show his constituents that he was active in their interests.[6]

By the beginning of August many people in Cork were taking flight. Often they moved semi-permanently to tourist hotels at either end of Cork county. Others took refuge with relatives in other parts of the country. Some even came to stay in the hotels overlooking the beaches in Youghal. It was a sensible reaction. Daniel Defoe in *A Journal of the Plague Year*, his classic account of the Great

Plague which devastated London in 1665, concludes baldly that 'the best physic against the plague is to run away from it'. Defoe was writing half a century after the event but he had studied contemporary accounts and had an extraordinarily acute sense of how people responded to the threat of disaster and disease. He says that many people had felt fatalistically that they might survive in London or die on their way to supposed safety and this was anyway all in God's hands. He wrote that this inertia 'kept thousands in the town whose carcasses went into the great pits by cartloads; and who, if they fled from the danger, had, I believe, been safe from the disaster'.[7] The doctors in Cork three hundred years later argued that the polio virus spread so swiftly that it did not matter much if people stayed in their houses or moved elsewhere. But this is not quite true, since most of those who were crippled by the disease lived in or near Cork city. Running away – even from so inexorable an enemy as the polio virus – had a lot to recommend it.

Since the start of the epidemic the doctors and Cork Corporation had recommended that children be kept off the streets. It was easy enough to stop circuses or close swimming baths. Irritation was expressed by almost everybody in an official position at the sight of children congregating in public. In Dublin Mrs Tom Barry, the head of the Irish Red Cross Society, offered the services of members to help the over-stretched doctors and nurses. She also asked branches of the Red Cross to stop during the epidemic the traditional fund-raising method of getting children to collect waste paper. She added that she 'was often horrified to see small children at all hours of the night dragging dirty sacks through the streets and

275

salvaging filthy paper from dustbins'.[8] For all the hysteria about spreading the disease, there was no suggestion that pubs, then as now the main social gathering place in Ireland, should be closed to prevent the spread of the virus.

Dr Saunders was aware that it was not children alone who caught polio or spread the virus. But he was prepared to go along with the myth that adults were invulnerable to catching it or could not be carriers, to avoid being forced into implementing measures of quarantine which he thought were useless. A Gaelic football match was to take place in Dublin's Croke Park on 7 August and he was under pressure to have it postponed so as to prevent an exodus of thousands of Cork people to Dublin to watch it. Instead he and the Chief Medical Officer for Dublin asked the GAA, which oversaw the sport, to 'make an appeal that no person under 14 years should make the journey to Dublin on Sunday'.[9] As we have seen, the doctors' decision led to a torrent of abusive mail to the Department of Health accusing it of negligently allowing polio-stricken sports fans from Cork to infect the people of Dublin. Unfortunately, Cork won the match against Kildare and was in both the Gaelic football and hurling finals, also be played in Dublin. This time around the General Council of the GAA decided to postpone the matches until the epidemic was over.

There is a monotony about the way in which the doctors explained the mechanics of the epidemic and the inability of people in Cork to understand the process by which they were all catching the virus. The popular attitude towards the epidemic, whether it be in Cork, Chicago or New York, had been conditioned by centuries of epidemics such as that so graphically described by Defoe. Cork was a highly democratic city and local councillors expected frequent meetings with the doctors to be told what was going on. At a meeting of the Cork Country Health Committee on 14 August Dr McCarthy made the less than comforting comment that polio 'was working its way through the child population; unfortunately adults were affected also'. When adults did get it and were paralysed then the virus was more virulent than among children. He said there were some small optimistic signs of a reduction in the number of cases.

Dr McCarthy repeated his mantra that the epidemic was mild and was mainly affecting better-off children. A member of the committee asked him if excursions to places like Courtmacsherry, a seaside resort and my mother's birthplace, on the coast of West Cork could not be stopped. Others wondered why people would be suddenly struck down forty miles from the city and how the virus had got there. A member of the Dáil called E. Cotter, said it was being 'mooted that the disease is being cloaked in Cork city'. Refugees from Cork were not unwelcome in all areas. Another member of the Dáil from Crosshaven said the town had 'received many children from Cork' and was 'delighted to welcome them if they could help the children escape the disease'.

Dr McCarthy patiently explained that polio was a difficult disease to trace, though every lead was investigated. People would explain its spread by saying: 'My child was playing with Mrs Brown's child.' But they seldom knew exactly who was the carrier. He knew of cases where a child had caught polio though he or she had never been to Cork or within twenty-five miles of the city in his or her whole life. 'The healthiest people could be carriers of the disease, innocent carriers because there was no means of detecting its presence in them as could be done with diphtheria,' he said.[10] He thought that children should be vaccinated during the winter months if the Department of Health could obtain the vaccine. It never seems to have occurred to the doctors in Cork or the Department of Health to do what was being done in Chicago that summer and combat the epidemic by mass vaccinations. It was probably too late to go for this option by the summer of 1956 and, in any case, vaccine was not available in sufficient quantities.

A week later a younger doctor was more open and less optimistic about the waning of the disease. Dr P. Fitzpatrick, an assistant to Dr Saunders, was asked at a Corporation meeting on 21 August if it was premature to say that the peak of the epidemic had passed. It turned out that he did indeed think it was too early for such an optimistic assumption. He said that the worst of the epidemic was usually between the thirty-second and thirty-sixth weeks of the year.[11] 'It is premature to say we have passed the peak. We are slowly passing through it. Until another fortnight it is premature to say we have passed the worst'.[12] Other medical workers, such as Maureen O'Sullivan, the Red Cross nurse, thought highly of Dr Fitzpatrick and believed he did much of the effective work in City Hall though he was without an assistant.[13] By now 158 cases had been diagnosed, which going by Dr Saunders's multiple of up to two hundred for undiagnosed cases meant that as many as 31,600 people could have been infected by the polio virus. The death rate among those who had been paralysed was less than 1 per cent, compared to a death rate of 27.4 per cent in the epidemic of 1942 and 1943, when 133 people had died out of 487 diagnosed. This was the only epidemic in Ireland for which figures were available. In epidemics in other countries the average death rate was about 10 per cent. Looking to the future, Dr Saunders said that, since there was obviously no question of returning to the insanitary and unhygienic conditions which had once prevented epidemics, the only solution was an effective vaccine.

Going by the official figures, Dr Saunders and Dr McCarthy were right in thinking that the epidemic was ebbing by the middle of August when forty-seven people were diagnosed as having polio over the previous two weeks. Another thrity-nine caught it over the next three weeks.[14] But the virus was not disappearing or running out of victims as fast as the sudden dearth of news about polio in the papers might have suggested. Probably the growing international notoriety of the epidemic in August and September reinforced the Irish instinct, very strong in the 1950s, to keep bad news from strangers.

The doctors in charge of counter-measures, keeping to the same course they had followed since the epidemic began at the end of June, sounded far less frightened than the rest of the population. They remained numb to the terror it was creating. Dr McCarthy said that national schools might be closed for three weeks in areas where there had been cases of polio. But there would be no general closure because this 'would paralyse the ordinary social life of the community'. They gave permission for schools to be reopened for children over the age of ten but not for children who were younger. None of this was popular with parents or school managers or the Catholic

279

Church, which was in charge of the school system. They pointed out the difficulty of administering schools that were half closed and half open. One mother in Cork wondered why schools were to open when cinemas and swimming baths were still shut. She wrote: 'Altogether our children have had a poor summer – no swimming, no pictures, no sunshine – nothing but the backyard for many a little prisoner. They are in no shape now to face infection and for them all I put in a mother's plea.' Despite these reservations the Department of Education ordered school managers to reopen schools to children over ten.[15]

In one of the last newspaper references to the epidemic in the *Irish Times* on 20 September Dr McCarthy had another optimistic outburst. He said the outbreak 'appears to have run its course in Cork city. The indications are that it is moving away very slowly. It was a comparatively light form of the disease. In fact by comparison with the grave ones it is a trifling epidemic.' Just over a week later on 29 September I was diagnosed by Dr Gowen as having caught polio. A day or so later my father greeted my brother Andrew, bowed over and stumbling with fever, off the train from Dublin and he joined me in St Finbarr's.

The epidemic was petering out in the autumn of 1956 as was expected. Polio was, after all, called 'the summer plague'. But it did not entirely disappear and the virus continued its attacks well into the next year. Dr O'Callaghan agrees that the peak of the disease was in August and September, but 'there were a trickle of patients up to March and April'.[16] At the time I was admitted to hospital the medical system in Cork could scarcely cope with the numbers of victims. The doctors did not admit this publicly. But in a private message to the Board of Public Assistance on 24 September Dr Goold and the matron at St Finbarr's said 'the sisters and domestic staff have worked well under appalling conditions'.[17] The old North Infirmary in Cork had been reopened to take polio patients for whom there was no room elsewhere. At the end of August Dr St John O'Connell was asked to provide two hundred beds at Guarranebraher for victims of polio. He was aghast and responded that 'it would be impossible for him to provide adequate treatment for 200 bed patients, a large number of whom required serious operations'.[18]

Government resources were limited. Even hiring an extra surgeon for three months at Gurranebraher required the assent of the Minister of Health.[19] Pauline Kent, the psysiotherapist who looked after me, complains to this day about the miserable level of pay she received at the time. Low pay and the obvious dangers of the job may explain the difficulty in recruiting nurses. Both at Gurranebraher and the North Infirmary the matrons were finding it very difficult to replace nurses who left or to find new ones.[20] Overall, however, the health service worked well or at least no worse than in the rest of Western Europe. The epidemic had broken out just too soon for it to be stopped by the Salk vaccine as would have happened if it had been delayed another year. But the Department of Health was probably right in congratulating itself on setting up three regional centres which specialised in polio without which 'the epidemic would have been far more serious'.[21] Overall it found that in 1956 there had been 220 diagnosed cases of polio in Cork, out of a total of 499 in Ireland of whom twenty died. This means that over 50,000 people had been attacked by the virus. Most never realised they had ever had polio. Dr O'Callaghan said that in later years she would see people in Cork 'with a dropped foot and wonder if their muscles had been affected without them knowing why'.

The polio virus always caused unpleasant surprises. Early in the twentieth century specialists were confident that they were close to discovering an antidote. In the event an effective vaccine was not discovered for half a century. For decades it was not known how people caught polio, what exactly happened when the virus entered the body and why it was able to inflict such damage. After 1955, inoculation with the Salk vaccine and later with the Sabin vaccine rapidly eradicated the disease in the US and Europe. Today it survives mainly in Africa. The World Health Organisation was frustrated in its effort to eliminate polio entirely because people in Islamic states in northern Nigeria at first rejected the vaccine on the grounds that it might be part of a plot by the US to render Muslim men infertile.

But the legacy of polio turned out to be more menacing than appeared likely when it was finally brought under control in the 1950s and 1960s. It is not just that those who were crippled at the time remain crippled. There was a further nasty twist. Over the last thirty years survivors of the disease discovered that there was an unexpected additional price they had to pay in the form of post-polio syndrome. Forty years or more after they caught the disease, many victims found that their muscles were weakening and they suffered easily from exhaustion. Some even suspected that the polio virus might have mysteriously reawakened somewhere deep in their spines. It gradually became clear to hundreds of thousands of survivors of polio that their illness, devastating though it was at the time, also had an unpleasant sequel which struck them as they reached middle age.

The assault of the polio virus on the motor neurons controlling the muscles was always ferocious but seldom wholly successful. In most cases enough motor neurons, although diminished in number and in a battered condition, were able to continue operating the muscles. David Bodian had discovered in the 1940s that there had to be a very high casualty rate – not less than 60 per cent – among the motor neurons controlling a particular muscle for it to begin to lose its strength. The Canadian neurophysiologist Alan McComas discovered fifty years later that muscles believed unaffected had frequently lost 40 per cent of their controlling motor neurons. In cases of paralytic polio all muscles were affected and suffered damage. As the years passed the surviving motor neurons began to die off at an unexpectedly young age because of the damage inflicted long ago by the virus. They die young because, depleted in number, they are compelled to carry out the functions of motor neurons killed off by the original disease. Death comes because they are chronically overworked. The motor neurons sending messages to the muscles are already far less numerous than they would be in the body of someone who never caught polio. These extra casualties caused by overwork may push the overall death rate among them past the crucial 60 per cent mark, leading to the return of old disabilities or the development of new ones.[22] This is known as post-polio syndrome and it is bad news for anybody like myself who suffered from polio fifty years ago. It also means that the 50,000 or so who caught the virus in Cork then but apparently suffered no ill effects may now for the first time be suffering the symptoms of polio. In most cases they are probably unaware why they are so easily fatigued or have difficulty in walking. It would be difficult to prove the reason why they suffer from these surprising weaknesses. Most polio victims were never diagnosed. Of those that were treated almost no medical records survived past the 1960s. The medical authorities thought the disease was conquered and had done all the harm it could do.

The epidemic in Cork was a strange prelude to the years in which Ireland became a modern and developed country, whose success is studied by other countries emerging from the Third World. While researching this book I was repeatedly struck by the fact that few people in Cork or anywhere else understood the grim mechanics of the disease. They almost invariably assumed that it was the result of poverty and lack of development. The idea that progress, the development of clean water and sewage disposal might make people more vulnerable to a crippling disease never occurred to them. My parents certainly never understood that Brook Lodge behind its ivy-covered walls was a more dangerous place to live in the summer of 1956 when it came to polio than the most insanitary back streets of Cork city. Claud and Patricia were very strong-willed and were difficult to deflect from what they wanted to do. They also had the fatalistic attitude to illness against which Defoe warned so eloquently. Otherwise they might never have returned from London to Ireland when they did.

At the height of the epidemic in August the Papal Nuncio in Ireland, the Most Reverend Dr Levama, said it was 'necessary to salvation that people should suffer'. Insensitive though this sounds, it is to the credit of the Nuncio that he was speaking at a conference on the rehabilitation of people crippled by polio.[23] Nine years before the epidemic in Cork, Albert Camus had published his novel *The Plague*, a fictional account of a bubonic plague in Oran in Algeria in the 1940s. An allegory about the occupation of France by Germany, it is certainly the best-known European book about an epidemic published in the twentieth century. As an account of the spread of a terrifying disease, with hundreds dying every day, it is less convincing than Defoe, sometimes comically so. Despite the plague which kills hundreds every day people in Oran still frequent cafés, restaurants and even the opera where the lead singer actually expires on stage. (The inability of Camus to imagine a world without such amenities may unintentionally illuminate the lack of vigour in the French resistance to the German occupation.) The narrator has the prosaic thought, as Oran celebrates victory over the plague, that 'one learns in the midst of such tribulations, namely that there is more in men to admire than to despise'.

The last sentence of the book predicts that 'the day will come when, for the instruction or misfortune of mankind, the plague will rouse its rats and send them to die in some well-contented city'.[24] No doubt Camus was speaking of authoritarian governments rather than disease. In fact, polio may be one of the last of the plagues for which there was no cure which swept across Europe for thousands of years up to the middle of the twentieth century. It differed from other diseases because it crippled rather than killed. As a killer it never compared with cholera, typhus, malaria, yellow fever or consumption, but it carried an extra charge of fear because like leprosy and smallpox it disfigured and disabled the living. Aids is the only disease in the last half-century to create comparable terror. Polio existed in epidemic form for less than seventy years. Its conquest was one of the great achievements of the twentieth century. Before an effective vaccine was discovered nothing could be done to stop it. It inflicted and continues to inflict great suffering among its surviving victims. Very occasionally well-meaning people suggested to me as a child that sufferings built character and endurance. Even at the age of seven or eight I suspected I had acquired these supposed benefits at an excessive price.

Endnotes

One

1. Claud Cockburn, *View from the West* (London: MacGibbon & Kee 1961) p. 152.
2. Interview with John Gowen 24 June 1999.
3. Interview with Shirley Arbuthnot 15 August 2003.
4. Claud Cockburn op. cit. pp. 149–50.
5. Interview with Bessie O'Callaghan 16 August 2003.
6. 'County Home Indoor Register', information provided by Southern Health Board under Freedom of Information Act 6 November 2003.
7. Interview with Kay Long's younger brother Alan 25 March 2004.
8. Interview with Pauline Kent, my physiotherapist, 1 July 1999.
9. Interview with Andrew Cockburn 26 August 2003.
10. Claud Cockburn op. cit. p. 151.
11. Interviews with Kathleen O'Callaghan 2 July 1999 and 18 August 2002.
12. *Cork Examiner* 8 August 1956.
13. *Cork Examiner* 22 August 1956.

14. Claud Cockburn op. cit. p. 146.
15. Claud Cockburn op. cit. p. 147.
16. J. G. Lockhart, *Life of Scott* (London: Merill & Baker 1837) vol. 1 p. 12.
17. Michael B. A. Oldstone, *Viruses, Plagues and History* (Oxford University Press 1998) p. 95.
18. Tony Gould, *A Summer Plague: Polio and Its Survivors* (New Haven and London: Yale University Press 1995) pp. 3–28.
19. Interview with Kitty Lee 24 June 1999.
20. Claud Cockburn op. cit. pp. 148–9.

Two

1. Letter to Department of Health, National Archives, Dublin, B132/308, 4 August 1956.
2. Letter to Department of Health, National Archives, Dublin, B132/308, 27 August 1956.
3. Letter to Department of Health, National Archives, Dublin, B132/308, 10 August 1956.
4. Interview with Danny Murphy 26 June 1999.
5. Interview with John Creedon 25 June 1999.
6. Letter to Department of Health, National Archives, Dublin, B132/308, 7 September 1956.
7. Telegrams to Department of Health, National Archives, Dublin, B132/308, 26 July 1956 and 30 July 1956.
8. Ministerial Statement from Department of Health, National Archives, Dublin, B132/308, 30 July 1956.
9. Letter to Department of Health, National Archives, Dublin, B132/308, 8 August 1956.
10. *Cork Examiner* 25 July 1956.

11. Interview with Kathleen O'Callaghan 18 August 2003.
12. Letter to Department of Health, National Archives, Dublin, B132/308, 31 August 1956.
13. Interviews with Pauline Kent 1 July 1999 and 17 August 2003.
14. *Cork Examiner* 15 August 1956.
15. Interview with Kathleen O'Callaghan 2 July 1999.
16. Interview 26 March 2004 with patient, who did not want his name published, from near Fermoy who spent three weeks in St Finbarr's in 1956. Only the muscles of his throat were affected.
17. Interview with Andrew Cockburn 26 August 2003.
18. Claud Cockburn, *View from the West* (London: MacGibbon & Kee 1961) pp. 152–4.
19. Richard L. Bruno, *The Polio Paradox* (New York: Warner Books 2002) pp. 20–37. Details about the polio virus in this section are drawn from Bruno, Gould and Oldstone op. cit.
20. Memorandum from Department of Health, National Archives, Dublin B132/308, 15 July 1955.

Three

1. Interview with Anne O'Sullivan 30 March 2004.
2. Interviews with Maureen O'Sullivan 27 June 1999 and 29 August 2004.
3. Claud Cockburn, *View from the West* (London: MacGibbon & Kee 1961) pp. 154–5.
4. Memorandum to Department of Health, National Archieves, Dublin B132/308 17 August 1956.
5. Interview with Anne O'Sullivan 30 March 2004.
6. Interview with Pauline Kent 11 July 1999.

7. Interview with John Creedon 26 June 1999.
8. *Cork Examiner* 15 August 1956.
9. Interview with Kathleen O'Callaghan 2 July 1999.
10. *Irish Times* 25 July 1956.
11. Letter to Department of Health, National Archives, Dublin, A5/345, received 27 August 1956.
12. *The Times* 14 August 1956.
13. Letter to Department of Health, National Archives, Dublin, B132/316, 17 November 1956.
14. *Irish Times* 28 August 1956.
15. *Times* 10 August 1956.
16. *Irish Times* 17 August 1956.
17. *Cork Examiner* 12 September 1956.
18. Interview with Kitty Lee 24 June 1999.
19. Patricia Cockburn, *Figure of Eight* (London: Chatto & Windus 1985) p. 223.
20. Interview with John Creedon 26 June 1999.
21. Cork Archives Institute, CP/C/A/20, Cork Corporation Minutes, 14 May 1957.
22. Cork Archives Institute, CP/C/A/20, Cork Corporation Minutes, 12 November 1957.
23. Interview with Ted Tanner 3 April 2004.
24. Interview with Maureen O'Sullivan 27 June 1999.
25. Interview with Jim Costello 25 March 2004.

Four

1. Claud Cockburn, *Crossing the Line* (London: MacGibbon & Kee 1958) p. 204.
2. Interview with Dick Cunningham 29 March 2004.

Five

1. Sidney C. H. Cheung, 'Mystery and Memory Behind the Colonial Shift', Department of Anthropology, the Chinese University of Hong Kong, http://www.asa2000.anthropology.ac.uk/cheung/cheung.html
2. *Colombo Advertiser* 2 July 1907.
3. Andrew Cockburn, 'Waiting for China', Condé Nast *Traveler* magazine August 1993, pp. 90–122.
4. Interview with Bessie O'Callaghan 17 August 2003.
5. Mark Girouard, 'Newtown Anner, Co. Tipperary', *Country Life*, 8 September 1988. A masterly account of the marriage between Sir Thomas Osborne and Catherine Smith drawing on the Osborne papers.
6. *Memorials of Lady Osborne* vol. 1 edited by her daughter Mrs Osborne, 2 vols (Dublin: Hodges, Foster & Co. 1870) pp. 32–40.
7. Anna Phipps, Newtown Anner papers, Hatfield House, Herts., p. 7. This is an account of their early years in Ireland by Anna, Lady Osborne's younger sister, who lived at Newtown Anner before her marriage to a Colonel Phipps. It was later transcribed in 1924. Part of the account is written by Beatrice Phipps.
8. Anna Phipps op. cit., p. 3.
9. Anna Phipps op. cit., p. 8.
10. Anna Phipps op. cit., p. 4.
11. *Memorials* op. cit. p. 8, 5 November 1816.
12. *Memorials* op. cit. p. xi.
13. *Memorials* op. cit. pp. 32–40.
14. Anna Phipps op. cit. p. 6.

15. Anna Phipps op. cit. p. 14.
16. *Memorials* op. cit. pp. 122–7.
17. Mark Girouard, 'Newtown Anner, Co. Tipperary,' *Country Life*, 15 September 1988, p. 227.
18. 'Notes, written for Lady Blake by Aunt Anna (Phipps), Sister of Lady Osborne.' MS in possession of Shirley Murray (Arbuthnot), Myrtle Grove.
19. *Dictionary of National Biography*, pp. 373–4.
20. Newtown Anner papers, Hatfield.
21. Henry Bagenal, *The Life of Bernal Osborne*, Preface by Duke of St Albans, for private circulation (London: Bentley & Son 1884), pp. 313–14.

Six

1. Patricia Cockburn, *Figure of Eight* (London: Chatto & Windus 1985) p. 8.
2. Edith Blake, MS in her own handwriting, dated Bermingham House 7 October 1880. MS in possession of Shirley Murray (Arbuthnot), Myrtle Grove.
3. Edith Osborne, *Twelve Months in Southern Europe* (London: Chapman & Hall, 1876) p. 260.
4. The account of the rows within the Osborne family are all taken from Edith Blake's account written in 1880.
5. Patricia Cockburn op. cit. pp. 12–13. Interview with Shirley Murray (Arbuthnot) 15 August 2003.
6. *World* 24 August 1881.
7. *Clonmel Chronicle, Tipperary and Waterford Advertiser* 26 June 1880 has a full transcript of the petty sessions at Stradbally, Co. Waterford. See also *Freeman's Journal* 10 July 1880.

8. *Daily Gleaner* Jamaica 28 January 1891. Sir Henry must have been the source of the detailed information about his family background.
9. *World* 24 August 1881.
10. *St James's Gazette* 16 September 1880.
11. *St James's Gazette* 16 September 1880.
12. *New York Times* 11 November 1888.
13. Patricia Cockburn op. cit. p. 14.
14. *The Times* 28 November 1888.
15. *Colombo Advertiser* 2 July 1907.
16. Andrew Cockburn op. cit. has a full account of the relations of the Tung family and Sir Henry's period as Governor of Hong Kong based partly on talks with the Tung family.
17. *Cork Examiner* 20 November 1913.

Seven

1. Alexander Cockburn, *Corruptions of Empire* (London and New York: Verso 1987) p. 6.
2. Interview with Paddy Linehan 24 March 2004.
3. National Archives, Kew, CO 914/115, monthly confidential report 2 June 1921.
4. National Archives, Kew, CO 904/146, summaries of police reports 1 June 1921.

Eight

1. Marcus Tanner, *Ireland's Holy Wars: The Struggle for a Nation's Soul* (New Haven and London: Yale University Press, 2001.

2. Benedict Anderson, 'Selective Kinship', *Dublin Review*, No. 10, Spring 2003 pp. 5–29.
3. Interview with Virginia Keane 14 November 2003.
4. Lavinia Greacen, *J. G. Farrell: The Making of a Writer* (London: Bloomsbury 1999) pp. 223–4.
5. Claud Cockburn, *Crossing the Line* (London: MacGibbon & Kee 1958) p. 190.

Nine

1. Patricia Cockburn, *Figure of Eight* (London: Chatto & Windus 1985) pp. 26–9.
2. Rex Taylor, *Assassination: The Death of Sir Henry Wilson and the Tragedy of Ireland* (London: Hutchinson 1961) pp. 15–89.
3. The message dropped by Terry is preserved at Myrtle Grove.
4. Claud Cockburn, *Crossing the Line* (London: MacGibbon & Kee 1958) p. 9.
5. Patricia Cockburn, op. cit. pp. 65–6.

Ten

1. Claud Cockburn, *In Time of Trouble* (London: Hart-Davis 1956) p. 23.
2. Patricia Cockburn, *The Week* (London: MacDonald 1968) pp. 56–7.
3. Richard Ingrams, *Muggeridge* (London: Harper-Collins 1996) p. xi.
4. 'How *Private Eye* Shook Whitehall by naming C', Richard Norton-Taylor, *Guardian*, 16 February 2000.

5. Patrick Marnham, *The Private Eye Story* (London: Andre Deutsch 1982) pp. 94–5.

6. Claud Cockburn op. cit. p. 23.

7. Claud Cockburn op. cit. pp. 46–7.

8. Claud Cockburn op. cit. p. 54.

9. Douglas Hyde, *I Believed* (London: The Reprint Society, 1950).

10. *The Times* 17 December 1981.

Eleven

1. National Archives, Kew, KV2 546, 10 April 1924.

2. National Archives, Kew, KV2 555, 1 April 1940.

3. National Archives, Kew, KV 1555, 12 February 1951.

4. National Archives, Kew, KV2 1555, 29 June 1948.

5. National Archives, Kew, KV2 547, 1 September 1935.

6. National Archives, Kew, KV2 547, 24 September 1937.

7. National Archives, Kew, KV2 552a, 2 May 1939.

8. National Archives, Kew, KV2 548, 26 February 1937.

9. National Archives, Kew, KV2 546, 1933.

10. National Archives, Kew, KV2 546, 9 July 1933.

11. National Archives, Kew, KV2 546, 20 July 1933.

12. National Archives, Kew, KV2/546, 18 January 1934.

13. National Archives, Kew, KV2 546, 19 March 1934.

14. National Archives, Kew, KV2 548, 1937.

15. National Archives, Kew, KV2 546, 23 October 1933.

16. National Archives, Kew, KV2 546, 2 November 1933.

17. National Archives, Kew, KV2 554, 8 November 1945.

18. National Archives, Kew, KV2 548, 28 October 1935.

19. National Archives, Kew, KV2 547, 2 August 1934.

20. National Archives, Kew, KV2 552, 29 March 1938.

21. *Week* 23 September 1935.

22. National Archives, Kew, KV2 548, 4 March 1937.
23. National Archives, Kew, KV2 548, 24 November 1936.
24. National Archives, Kew, KV2 552, 17 October 1940.
25. National Archives, Kew, KV2 554, Special Branch 15 April and 13 May 1941.
26. National Archives, Kew, KV2 554, 13 June 1941.
27. National Archives, Kew, KV2 1554, 26 February 1943.
28. National Archives, Kew, KV2 1955, 8 September 1949.
29. *Daily Express* 9 September 1949.
30. National Archives, Kew, KV2 555, 3 November 1949.
31. National Archives, Kew, KV2 555, 11 April 1950.
32. National Archives, Kew, KV2 555, 12 February 1951.
33. RASPI (Russian State Archive for Social and Political History), Fund 495, OPIC 198, Item 1370, 28 May 1937.
34. RASPI, Fund 495, OPIC 198, Item 1370, R. Stewart 7 April 1937.
35. RASPI, Fund 495, OPIC 198, Item 1370, J. Shields 28 August 1936.
36. RASPI, Fund 495, OPIC 198, Item 1370, R. Stewart 7 April 1937.
37. RASPI, Fund 495, OPIC 298, Item 1370, J. Shields 28 August 1936.
38. National Archives, Kew, KV2 546, 26 April 1934.

Twelve

1. Fiona Wallace, 'The impact of the Cork polio epidemic on voluntary provision for the handicapped', MA thesis 1994 NUI, Department of History, University College Cork.
2. Interview with Kathleen O'Callaghan 2 July 1999.

3. Interview with Jim Costello 25 March 2004. Mr Costello is chairman of the Post Polio Syndrome Group.
4. Donal O'Donovan, letter 30 March 2004.
5. Interview with Shirley Murray (Arbuthnot) 15 August 2003.
6. Interview with Pauline Kent 17 August 2003.
7. Interview with Leon Berger 7 October 2004. Mr Berger is writing the biography of Michael Flanders.
8. Tony Gould, *A Summer Plague: Polio and Its Survivors* (New Haven and London: Yale University Press 1995) pp. 90–91.
9. Michael B. A. Oldstone, *Viruses, Plagues and History* (Oxford University Press 1998) p. 91.
10. *Irish Times* 24 August 1956.
11. Gould op. cit. p. 161.
12. Oldstone op. cit. p. 91.

Thirteen

1. Interview with Paddy Linehan 24 March 2004.
2. Terence Browne, *Ireland: A Social and Political History* (Glasgow: Fontana Paperbacks 1981) p. 241.
3. Interview with John Gowen 24 June 1999.
4. Browne op. cit. p. 186.
5. Interview with Pauline Kent 17 August 2003.
6. *Irish Times* 17 August 1956.
7. *Cork Examiner* 22 August 1956.
8. Fiona Wallace, 'The impact of the Cork polio epidemic on voluntary provision for the handicapped', MA thesis 1994 NUI, Department of History, University College Cork, p. 32.

9. *Cork Examiner* 22 August 1956.

10. *Irish Times* 9 August 1956.

11. Interview with Maura McGuane 2 July 1999.

12. Interview with Donal Walsh 20 August 2003.

13. *Irish Times* 9 August 1956.

14. National Archives, Dublin, DH B132/308.

15. Fiona Wallace op. cit. p. 41.

16. Interview with Kathleen O'Callaghan 18 August 2003.

17. Thomas Dormandy, *The White Death: A History of Tuberculosis* (London and New York: Hambledon & London 1999) pp. 240–1.

18. Fiona Wallace op. cit. p. 38, citing *Evening Echo* 14 July 1956.

19. J. G. Lockhart, *Life of Scott* (London: Merrill & Baker, 1837) Vol. 1, pp. 10–15).

20. Interview with Anne O'Sullivan 30 March 2004.

21. Interview with Professor John Hall 30 June 1999.

22. Claud Cockburn, *View from the West* (London: MacGibbon & Kee 1961) p. 155.

23. Richard L. Bruno, *The Polio Paradox* (New York: Warner Books 2002) pp. 38–59.

24. Oldstone, *Viruses, Plagues and History* (Oxford University Press 1998) p. 95.

25. Interview with Professor John Hall 30 June 1999.

26. *Cork Examiner* 22 August 1956.

27. *Cork Examiner* 15 August 1956.

28. Interview with Maureen O'Sullivan 26 September 1999.

29. *Irish Times* 9 August 1956.

30. Richard L. Bruno op. cit. p. 42.

31. Interview with Mary O'Riordan 9 August 2004.

32. Interview with Dr Kathleen O'Callaghan 18 August 2003.

33. *Cork Examiner* 16 July 1956.
34. *Cork Examiner* 16 July 1956.
35. *Cork Examiner* 12 July 1956.
36. *Cork Examiner* 16 July 1956.
37. *Cork Examiner* 21 July 1956.
38. Fiona Wallace op. cit. p. 45, citing interview with John Bermingham, a councillor on 1 December 1992.
39. *Cork Examiner* 24 July 1956.
40. *Cork Examiner* 27 July 1956.
41. *Cork Examiner* 28, 30 July 1956.

Fourteen

1. Interviews with Pat Field 31 March 2004 and Helena Chapman 3 April 2004.
2. *Cork Examiner* 8 August 1956.
3. *Cork Examiner* 9 August 1956.
4. *Cork Examiner* 11 August 1956.
5. National Archives, Dublin, Department of Health, B132/308, letter 31 August 1956.
6. National Archives, Dublin, Department of Health, B132/308, 11 August 1956.
7. Daniel Defoe, *A Journal of the Plague Year*, first published in 1722 (London: Penguin edition 2003) p. 190.
8. *Cork Examiner* 20 July 1956.
9. *Cork Examiner* 1 August 1956.
10. *Cork Examiner* 15 August 1956.
11. *Cork Examiner* 22 August 1956.
12. *Cork Examiner* 22 August 1956.
13. Interview with Maureen O'Sullivan 22 August 1999.
14. Cork Corporation Public Health Committee, CP/C/CM/PH/A/35, p. 185.

15. Fiona Wallace, 'The impact of the Cork polio epidemic on voluntary provision for the handicapped', MA thesis 1994 NUI, Department of History, University College Cork, p. 54.
16. Interview with Kathleen O'Callaghan 2 July 1999.
17. Cork Archives Institute, CC/CCBA, p. 9, 24 September 1956.
18. Cork Archives Institute, CC/CCBA, p. 8, 27 August 1956.
19. National Archives, Dublin, Department of Health, A5/345, 15 July 1956.
20. National Archives, Dublin, Department of Health, A5/345, 17 August 1956.
21. Medical Year Book 1956.
22. Richard L. Bruno, *The Polio Paradox* (New York: Warner Books 2002) p. 118.
23. *Cork Examiner* 11 August 1956.
24. Albert Camus, *The Plague* first published in 1947 (London: Penguin edition 2001) pp. 237–8.

Acknowledgements

Many people have contributed to writing this book. I was six when I caught polio so my memories of the epidemic are vivid but episodic. I have therefore relied heavily on the recollections of doctors, nurses and victims for details of what happened. I was pleasantly surprised to find that they confirmed almost everything that I recalled.

I am also very grateful for the help given me in tracing the history of my family from the beginning of the nineteenth century. Fortunately many of my ancestors were copious correspondents and kept their letters or wrote for the newspapers even when they were serving as policemen or army officers. A gratifying number also wrote books. They also had the habit, useful for the historian, of pasting into large albums many press clippings about themselves and their times which would not otherwise have survived.

I am particularly thankful to my cousin Shirley Arbuthnot for showing me some of the Blake papers. Mark Girouard was very helpful in talking about the Osbornes and showing me his writings about the family. Robin Harcourt Williams, Librarian and Archivist to the Marquess of Salisbury, found a fascinating diary in the Osborne papers kept at Hatfield House. Barry McLoughlin suggested that I write to MI5 asking for the file on my father which turned out to be twenty-six volumes long. He also identified Claud's Comintern file in the Russian State Archive for Social and Political History in Moscow.

The events described in the book are long enough ago that some of those who were the most helpful such as Kitty Lee, who looked after me for so long, and Paddy Linehan, with his intimate knowledge of events in Youghal, have died since they were interviewed.

I would like to thank the following in particular for their help: Colin Anson, Shirley Arbuthnot, Prof. Dick Barry, Leon Berger, Peggy Brennan, Helena Chapman, Alexander Cockburn, Andrew Cockburn, Jim Costello, John Creedon, Alan Crosbie, Dick Cunningham, Pat Field, Dr John Gowen, Prof. John Hall, Clara Hughes, Sally Keane, Virginia Keane, Pauline Kent, Alan Long, Maura McGuane, Danny Murphy, Donal O'Donovan, Bessie O'Callaghan, Kathleen O'Callaghan, Mary O'Riordan, Anne O'Sullivan, Maureen O'Sullivan (Post-Polio Syndrome Group), Maureen O'Sullivan (formerly of the International Committee of the Red Cross), Ted Tanner, Evelyn Wainwright, Donal Walsh.

I would like to thank Dan Franklin for being such an enthusiastic and intelligent editor and David Miller for his wise advice and assistance.

My brother Andrew read all the manuscript and my brother Alexander read part of it. Both made useful critical comments. Lucretia Stewart played a key role in getting the project underway. My wife Janet selflessly read through each chapter as it was written offering morale-boosting support and making many valuable suggestions. She also put up with the author spending half his time writing this book and the rest of it in Iraq before, during and after the US invasion.

Index

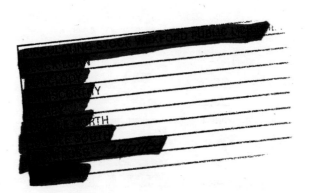